Disease, Diagnosis and Decisions

Disease, Diagnosis and Decisions

GRAHAM W. BRADLEY BSc PhD FRCP
Consultant Physician and Clinical Director of Medicine,
South Kent Hospitals, UK

JOHN WILEY & SONS
Chichester · New York · Brisbane · Toronto · Singapore

Other Wiley Editorial Offices

John Wiley & Sons, Inc., 605 Third Avenue,
New York, NY 10158-0012, USA

Jacaranda Wiley Ltd, G.P.O. Box 859, Brisbane,
Queensland 4001, Australia

John Wiley & Sons (Canada) Ltd, 22 Worcester Road,
Rexdale, Ontario M9W 1L1, Canada

John Wiley & Sons (SEA) Pte Ltd, 37 Jalan Pemimpin #05-04,
Block B, Union Industrial Building, Singapore 2057

Library of Congress Cataloging-in-Publication Data

Bradley, Graham W.
    Disease, diagnosis and decisions / Graham W. Bradley.
        p. cm.
    Includes bibliographical references and index.
    ISBN 0 471 93929 3
        1. Medicine—Decision making. 2. Diagnosis. 3. Medicine—
    Philosophy. 4. Probability. I. Title.
        [DNLM: 1. Philosophy. Medical. 2. Diagnosis. 3. Logic.
    4. Decision Making. W 61 B811d 1992]
    R723.5.B67   1992
    610—dc20
    DNLM/DLC
    for Library of Congress   93-17986
                                                                  CIP

British Library Cataloguing in Publication Data

A catalogue record for this book is available from the British Library

ISBN 0 471 93929 3

Typeset in 11/13pt Palatino by Dobbie Typesetting Ltd, Tavistock, Devon
Printed and bound in Great Britain by Biddles Ltd, Guildford, Surrey

To Joyce, Dylan, Davy and Helen
for the loss of the shared evenings
and weekends which can
never be recaptured

Contents

Preface

Medical students soon learn that the practice of medicine is far from straightforward: there are difficult choices to be made and risks to take. As a young medical student, steeped in anatomical, physiological and biochemical knowledge, ready and keen to apply this knowledge to my future patients, I was somewhat disappointed when the ageing—but no doubt wise—Professor of Surgery spent all of his first lecture showing how the treatment of blisters had changed over the years. It seemed to be either mandatory or contra-indicated to puncture blisters depending on which decade you lived in. Apart from leading to a lifelong distrust of the words 'mandatory' and 'contra-indicated', this shook my confidence. If we didn't know how to treat blisters what hope was there for the treatment of more complicated conditions? This was my first encounter with medical uncertainty and the unease which it produced stayed with me for some time. It had the positive effect of triggering an interest in the reasons for uncertainty and in ways by which it can be reduced. This book arises out of this interest and is intended for anyone who has felt uncomfortable practising medicine when the cause of illness is uncertain and the response to treatment unpredictable.

Why is there so much uncertainty about the diagnosis and management of disease if modern medicine is based on scientific principles? We associate science with consistency and certainty; the complex technology which modern society relies so heavily upon seems to attest to this. What must seem to many to be a paradox of medical science is that whilst there have been striking developments in medicine, there are also large areas which remain poorly understood. We can transplant hearts but cannot cure the common cold. Even when active treatment for illness is available we often do not know the optimum management and cannot predict the outcome, even in statistical terms, with any degree of accuracy. This leads to wide variation in practice in the same health care system, let alone between health care systems in different countries.

There are, I believe, two reasons for this uncertainty. The first arises from the limitations of classical science when applied to complex systems. The physics, chemistry and biology I had been taught at medical school was based on Newtonian principles with cause and effect leading to a world which is certain and predictable. Since basic science is based on these principles, this is still the approach taken in medical schools today. The principles have been enormously successful when applied to a wide spectrum of natural phenomena including many relevant to medical practice, but they fail to deal adequately with complex non-linear systems such as the whole human body. Not only are there practical difficulties in establishing the current physiological, biochemical and even anatomical condition of our patients, but also there are many factors which can influence the outcome of proposed treatment with considerable potential for interaction. Whilst it is possible in principle to understand and measure all these factors, in practice some are poorly understood and many cannot be measured. Inevitably, therefore, a person's response to disease and its treatment is not always predictable with the high degree of certainty we would like to see.

This difficulty in predicting the response of complex systems applies to many physical systems such as the weather. In contrast, the second basic limitation is peculiar to the problems of obtaining information from a living organism. Not only are biological systems more complex, but they are also more difficult to study; the mysteries of life can only be fully understood by examining living organisms, and, in consequence, the types of experiments which can be performed are restricted. The effect of disease on morbid anatomy, both macroscopic and microscopic, can only give a limited understanding. This is not to deny the importance of such studies, but a full understanding of disease processes can only be obtained in living organisms, and it goes without saying that management of disease must be studied in live people.

This raises both ethical and practical problems. The simplest and most revealing experiments are often unethical: for example, we do not really know the advantages of surgery for many cancers, but a prospective randomized trial of surgery against no action would be regarded as quite unacceptable. There are practical problems too: the confirmation of a small but, nevertheless, useful effect of a drug, requires a study involving a large number of people and this can be difficult to organize. A number of centres may need to participate, thus presenting problems of standardization, management and collection of accurate data. Not surprisingly, therefore, much of the data published in the medical literature either fails to ask a useful question or fails to answer the question asked. Some of these problems are discussed in the chapter on limitations of statistical methods.

Since modern medicine is generally regarded as a scientific subject based on Newtonian principles, the approach taken in this book is to look at the limitations of the scientific method when applied to the diagnosis and management of disease. Some people would regard this as a narrow approach. Undoubtedly the practice of medicine involves more than the application of the scientific method to medical problems, since health is not just the absence of disease, but something which involves a positive attitude to life both physically and mentally. Nevertheless, there can be no doubt that the scientific approach to disease forms an important, and perhaps the most important, aspect of medicine. For this reason this book starts with an analysis of the meaning of disease and places this in an historical context. We shall see that the classification of medical conditons into categories called diseases was an important step in the evolution of medicine. Whilst medical practice is still a merger of 'art' and 'science' there can be no doubt that the application of the scientific method to medicine was the further crucial step which led to an explosive growth in our knowledge of illness and of our ability to deal with it.

We shall explore what is meant by the scientific method, but what do we mean by art in this context? Doctors often talk about the art of medicine and sometimes revel in the mystique surrounding this. Perhaps this goes back to the origin of medicine in religion and magic, but I would interpret the art of medicine as the process of making reasonable decisions in uncertain circumstances—a question of judgement involving a combination of knowledge, personal experience, common sense and humanity. Inevitably, there is a large subjective aspect to such decision making, but the degree of uncertainty can be reduced by using techniques described in this book.

The scientific approach has been so crucial to the development of medicine that I believe it is important to understand the nature of this approach and its limitations. In that the scientific process is essentially a rational process, it is inescapable that the rational way of thinking has determined the development of the scientific method. Both philosophers and psychologists have contributed to our understanding of the thinking process, but, since the study of psychology is a relatively recent development, it is the philosophers who have laid down the foundation of cognitive science. Philosophy is a discipline with which few medical students or doctors concern themselves, probably because of the lack of time rather than inclination, so I hope that the reader will find the chapter on philosophy, science and medicine both interesting and relevant. The debate concerning the relative importance of inductive and deductive reasoning is described, as well as the concept of causality which has been central to scientific thinking. Whilst modern medicine is based on the concept of cause and effect, science itself has moved forward into the less predictable world of quantum mechanics and chaos theory. These concepts are difficult to visualize and grasp, but chaos theory, which is introduced in this chapter, is particularly relevant to illness and medical practice.

The way we think must be relevant to the principles of the scientific approach. The hypothetico-deductive method, lucidly described by Peter Medawar[1] in his book, *Induction and Intuition in Scientific Thought*, emerges as the best description of the thinking process, and in this approach the concepts of inductive and deductive logic are merged. Observations lead to the generation of hypotheses from which, by a process of deduction, consequences can be derived which can then be put to the test. The hypothesis which withstands the rigour of testing is accepted as valid, at least for the time being. The process of hypothesis generation and testing is central to rational thinking and therefore relevant to the diagnostic process. Considerable work has been published on the use of hypothetico-deductive methods in diagnosis, and this is described in Chapter 3. Mention is also made of the observation, which must be apparent to everyone, that human beings are not always rational: whilst this could be regarded as a weakness rather than a strength, there is no doubt that intuitive reasoning is one of the highest human faculties. The difficulties encountered in developing computer diagnostic systems (Chapter 5) give further insight into human reasoning.

The diagnostic process starts with a thorough history taken from the patient and a relevant physical examination. Often this suffices to make a confident diagnosis, but the cause of a person's illness may remain uncertain without recourse to some investigation such as a blood test or radiological examination. There has been a rapid increase in the development of such investigations during this century helping enormously in the diagnosis and understanding of disease. However, many tests do not provide a precise diagnosis, although the result of a test should change the likelihood of a possible diagnosis, otherwise there would be little point in doing it. The question then raised is what is the likelihood of a possible diagnosis, given the clinical features and the result of a particular investigation. This leads us into a branch of statistics called conditional probability, the rules for which were laid down by Thomas Bayes. When Stephen Hawking[2] wrote *A Brief History of Time*, he was advised not to include any formulae for fear of frightening off potential readers. I have taken this risk with the chapter about Bayesian statistics, but I can assure the reader that the mathematics involved is elementary and the notation soon learned: the principles of Bayesian statistics are so fundamental to the correct interpretation of medical investigations that a little effort to understand the concepts is well worthwhile.

Even when the diagnosis is known, the best approach to the management of a problem may still be unclear. The chapter on decision analysis introduces methods which can be used to optimize decisions when there is a background of uncertainty. These techniques have been developed particularly for the business world. Whilst it is difficult to foresee the widespread introduction of these techniques into routine clinical practice, there are areas where they could be useful, particularly when the management options are well defined and the probable outcomes of various choices are known. One branch of decision analysis, utility analysis, allows the patient to participate in the decision making process; and another technique, cost effectiveness analysis, takes account of the economic aspects of health care. Both these are perceived to be of increasing importance in the modern world, but perhaps the most important message is that these techniques contain an element of gamble which doctors and patients should recognize and accept.

An understanding of statistics is increasingly important in medical practice and is obviously relevant to an exploration of uncertainty in medicine. There are many excellent texts on medical statistics and it would have been inappropriate to have included formal statistical analysis in this book. However, it does seem apt to highlight the limitations of statistics, particularly in relation to medical trials. The accuracy and relevance of such trials is important in forming a reliable factual base from which sensible decisions can be taken. Unfortunately, there are many pitfalls for the unwary in the use and interpretation of statistics, but even when used correctly, a large subjective aspect to the interpretation of statistical results remains. Some of these pitfalls, and the subjective nature of probability, are discussed in Chapter 7.

Despite increasing concern about variations in medical practice, the difficulties which are the root cause of this unsettling state of affairs are not generally taught at medical school. The aim of this book is to encourage medical students and doctors to analyse the reasons for uncertainty and to learn something of the techniques which are available to deal with this. This book covers a wide range of topics; no one person can be an expert in fields as diverse as philosophy, computers and statistics, and the reader should not be surprised to find that I am not an expert in any. My interest in these topics stems from a desire to explore the limits of medical science with a view to living more comfortably with uncertainty. More detailed coverage can be found in the suggested further reading at the end of each chapter and in the more specific references indicated in the text, which are given in full at the end of the book.

Problem solving in medicine consists of making adequate decisions with inadequate information, but doctors can take some comfort from the fact that they are not alone in their difficulties.

Similar problems are encountered by politicians, economists, judges and generals. As Denis Healey pointed out in his autobiography, 'Unpredictability and uncertainty play such an important role in both politics and economics that no practical politician should allow himself to be imprisoned in a single systematic theory or doctrine.' It is this process of judgement, by which sound decisions are made with imperfect information, which is regarded as the art of medicine. However successful the scientific approach is, it will never eliminate this subjective aspect of medical practice.

Acknowledgements

Any new book is based on the experience and publications of many people. To these I express my gratitude for their stimulus and expertise, particularly those authors acknowledged in the bibliography at the end of each chapter. It would have been impossible for me to write this without relying heavily on their scholarship.

Several friends and colleagues have encouraged me to write this book and have been kind enough to read and criticise early drafts. I am particularly indebted to Bob Kempson, Simon Kenwright, John Lines and Adrian Morris for their comments and suggestions. No doubt they agreed with some of what is written but no one would agree with all. The responsibility for the views expressed is entirely my own.

1

The Nature of Disease

'When I use a word it means just what I choose it to mean—neither more nor less.'

Humpty Dumpty
(Lewis Carroll—*Through the Looking Glass*)

INTRODUCTION

This book is about the origin and management of uncertainty in medical practice. Since the diagnosis and treatment of disease is central to medicine, we shall start by trying to define what is meant by the word. This is more difficult than it might appear to be at first sight, and resorting to a dictionary seems not to help: the *Concise Oxford Dictionary* defines disease as a morbid condition and morbid as indicative of disease. The origin of the word, as with so many words, has been lost in the sands of time, but we do know that the etymology is old French. Fortunately, for the purpose of this book, the origin of the word is irrelevant, but what do people mean by the term?

Campbell et al.[3] looked into this by reading out a list of common diagnostic terms to groups of medical and non-medical people. The participants were then asked whether they would regard the condition as a disease. Their responses are shown in Figure 1.1 from which some general conclusions can be drawn. First, doctors are more likely to call a medical condition a disease. Secondly, when the cause of illness is a known physical or chemical agent, the condition is less likely to be regarded as a disease. On the other hand, any illness due to a micro-organism

1

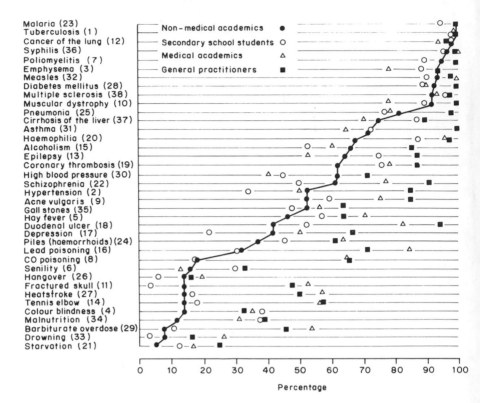

Figure 1.1 *Opinion of four groups as to whether the medical conditions shown should be regarded as diseases. The number after the medical condition indicates the order in which the questions were asked. From Campbell et al. (1979), with permission.*[3]

was considered to be a disease by the great majority of people. A third finding was that a medical condition was likely to be thought a disease if a doctor's contribution to the diagnosis was important.

It is clear from this that people mean different things by the word disease and use the term inconsistently. In a thorough analysis of the nature of disease, Reznek[4] argued that the use of the term is not closely related to the cause, progression or timing of the illness. The meaning of words often evolve with time and our concept of disease is certain to have been influenced by the evolution of medical knowledge over many centuries. In view of this, I have included a brief synopsis of medical history as the starting point of this book, and this is followed by a critical analysis of what, to me, is still the best practical definition of disease, despite its limitations.

SYNOPSIS OF MEDICAL HISTORY

Primitive Medicine

Mankind has always been subjected to ill-understood calamities of one kind or another, and early man saw the hand of some all powerful god, or gods, being involved. Gradually a class of men emerged who claimed special access to these gods and eventually, in the course of time, they became witch doctors or priests. It is hardly surprising that the manifestations of illness became their prerogative so medicine and religion became inseparable. Because doctors were also priests, in early Egyptian history medicine seemed surprisingly specialized. Each priest dealt with a different God and, therefore, concerned themselves with the disease said to be under the influence of their particular deity.

The first doctor to be mentioned by name was Imhotep, who, as well as being a statesman and physician to the king, was responsible for the building of the step pyramid of Sakharah. He lived about 3000 BC and in the course of time he was elevated to the rank of god. Some may say, with a touch of irony, the first of many.

In Greece, at a later period, the god of health and medicine was Apollo who was reported to have a son, Asclepius, referred to as the blameless physician. He suffered the wrath of Zeus and was killed by a thunderbolt but he was subsequently elevated to a god of medicine, perhaps the first example of patrimony in medicine. The cult of the serpent as a symbol of healing is associated with the name of Asclepius, although it came from Minoan civilization. The snake is still regarded as a medical emblem to this day.

Surgery

The practical management of injuries and surgical conditions such as broken bones and abscesses was evident from an early age in all cultures, but only in India was the surgeon considered to have superior status. In Western societies, partly due to the views of the influential Galen, who treated surgery with contempt, surgery was not considered to be a suitable career for a gentleman until the barber–surgeons split into their respective specialties. Nowadays, surgeons have a pre-eminent position in the ranking of status within the medical profession, but the early days were not easy. An early Babylonian king, Hammurabi, decreed that, 'If a doctor, in opening an abscess, shall kill the patient, his hands shall be cut off.' Surgery in the times of the Visigoths was no less exacting: any doctor allowing a patient to die through blood letting was delivered into the hands of grieving relatives to be dealt with as they felt appropriate. This robust approach certainly concentrates the mind; modern litigation-conscious medicine seems almost tame by comparison.

Surgery in these early days was held back by limited knowledge of anatomy. Dissection of human corpses was not allowed in most cultures, but in the Brahmian period of Indian medicine bodies could be examined so long as they had been placed in a basket and soaked in a river for seven days. Inevitably, this led to an emphasis on bones, joints, muscles and ligaments. Even Galen was not allowed to dissect human bodies, learning much of his anatomy by dissecting apes and pigs. Considering their limited anatomical knowledge and primitive utensils the type of surgery undertaken at this time was quite amazing. Excision of tumours, stitching wounds, incision of abscesses and even plastic surgery was undertaken in India during the Brahmian period (800 BC to 1000 AD). Plastic surgery was undertaken to fashion new noses from the cheek, an operation much in demand since the punishment for adultery was amputation of the nose. Even intestinal operations were performed in which an ingenious process of suturing was undertaken. Giant black ants were made to bite the edges of the wound together after which their bodies were cut off to form a primitive stitch.

Interest in anatomical knowledge began to flourish in the 15th and 16th century led by Renaissance artists such as Michelangelo, Dürer and Leonardo da Vinci, who were interested in drawing the body in proportion. The publication on the fabric of the human body by Vesalius (1514–64) in 1543 proved to be a major advance in our understanding and dissemination of anatomical knowledge. This work was notable for being based on his own observations rather than reiterating Galen's views and, consequently, surgery profited from this better understanding of anatomy. A major sensation was his demolition of the age-old fable that men had one rib fewer than women.

Following this improved knowledge of anatomy, significant advances were made in surgical technique and no-one did more for the reputation of surgery than Ambroise Paré (1510–90) who had the honour of being surgeon to four kings of France, earning himself the title of 'Father of Modern Surgery' in the process. But, even so, at the time of the French Revolution surgeons were still regarded as artisans rather than gentlemen, although Desault (1744–95) was respected particularly for his efforts to formalize training. What led to a quantum leap in status was the French Revolution, when it quickly became apparent that surgeons were more effective at dealing with the carnage of war than were the effete physicians. It was at this time that physicians became more practical in outlook and the dominance of Galen was finally laid to rest.

Two further major advances which revolutionized surgery, anaesthetics and antiseptics, are well known. Alcohol was used as a primitive anaesthetic not only in the Wild West of America but also, well before, in India. The soporific effects of the mandrake plant were known to the Assyrians, but other attempts at early anaesthesia were less appealing. They included pressure on the carotid arteries to induce unconsciousness, and bleeding the patient until insensible. The numbing effect of intense cold was also put to use by one of Napoleon's chief surgeons during the retreat from Moscow.

The dawn of modern anaesthesia began with Humphry Davy (1778–1829) who discovered the effect of both nitrous oxide and ether, but he did not pursue the matter. Horace Wells (1815–48) in Connecticut extracted teeth using nitrous oxide, but his first public demonstration was less than an outright success, and like so many medical men who made major discoveries which were not immediately accepted he became disillusioned, left medicine and took his own life. Morton (1819–68), who was present at Wells' demonstration, experimented with ether and gave a successful demonstration at the Massachusetts General Hospital in Boston in 1846. Anaesthesia was soon firmly established although Morton himself was virtually ostracized because, for commercial gain, he attempted to disguise ether as a new discovery.

Lister (1827–1912) was impressed with the advantages of anaesthesia, but horrified by the death toll resulting from infections which followed operations. Although microbes had not been discovered, it was becoming accepted that infection was due to some 'miasma' in the air, and Lister sought some chemical which might neutralize it. He found this in the work of a Manchester chemist named Calvert who had reported success in using carbolic acid to disinfect and deodorize sewage. In 1865 Lister first used carbolic acid on a compound fracture with a good result. On reading the work of Pasteur in the same year he realized that he was on the right lines. The concept of antisepsis was quickly established, and the subsequent step to asepsis led to further improvement in results and the birth of modern surgery.

Medical Paradigms

Alongside the early development of practical skills, physicians have not been slow to hypothesize as to the cause and cure of illness. Even the earliest of surgeons, those who made trephine holes in their patients' skulls using flints, almost certainly believed that they were releasing the malevolent demon. One suspects that the practice was apparently vindicated by the 'peace' found by most of their patients following this procedure, yet some survived as shown by new bone formation around the 'burr' hole seen in some skulls.

Anyone dealing with patients will know only too well how readily laymen can generate hypotheses to explain illness. Perhaps this is natural curiosity tempered by a fear of ill health, but the situation is not quite as bad as in Babylonia where everyone was regarded as an amateur physician. As reported in Heroditus' history, it was the custom to lay the sick in the street so that any passers-by could offer their opinion. There are times when even the modern physician is tempted to revert to this practice.

Whilst some philosophers have encouraged an empirical approach to knowledge, people seem to have difficulty in thinking without the framework of a working hypothesis. In the Brahmian period of Indian medicine the prevailing hypothesis was of three diverse forces controlling disease: phlegm originating above the heart, bile below the heart, and the spirit or air below the navel. If these are regarded anatomically as approximately correct, it says something about the diet of the time. A similar concept originated in Greece with the doctrine of four bodily humours: blood, phlegm, yellow bile, and black bile, the latter leading to the term melancholy (Greek for black bile) which is still in use. This system of medicine subsequently had the seal of approval from Galen.

Other cultures developed different conceptual frameworks of disease. Chinese medicine was strongly influenced by the dualistic cosmic theory of Yin and Yang. Literally, this refers to the two banks of a river, one in the shade and the other in the sun. Yang, the male principle, was active and light represented by the heavens, whereas Yin was dark, passive and female represented by the earth. The aim of medicine was to control the proportions. This led to an elaborate classification of disease in which most of the types listed were without firm foundation. In China, the doctrine of the pulse dominated medicine. The minimum time which was regarded as necessary to feel the pulse was ten minutes and the whole operation, given that there are several pulses to feel, could last three hours. It was thought that energy passed between certain well defined points in the body, and insertion of needles at these points adjusted the balance of Yin and Yang. This procedure of acupuncture is preferable to the alternative of moxibustion whereby cones, consisting of the leaves of the moxa plant, were placed at important points and ignited! Both these techniques are still in use in China.

Another dualistic concept was developed in relatively modern times by John Brown (1735–88) and became known as the Brunian system. This theory was an example of the vitalist backlash to the increasingly popular mechanistic view of medicine. In some respects vitalism—which was developed particularly in Montpellier in France—was a temporary reversion to the pneumona of the ancients. In the Brunian system life resulted from nervous forces responding to excitation to a variable extent and disease was a manifestation of either too much of it or too little. Two types of diseases were recognized, the sthenic (strong) and asthenic (weak), and the two main remedies for these were sedation and stimulation. John Brown's death was accelerated by the frequent use of his two main treatments, opium and alcohol!

An alternative tradition to the embryonic scientific method was the occult, with natural magic, as distinct from sorcery, being accepted by men of learning. Detailed rules were laid down to enable the magus to discover hidden sympathies and antipathies with a view to developing any practical use they might have. A key feature of this approach was the likeness of things, with like attracting like, the so-called doctrine of signatures. It was argued that the herb scorpius, by resembling the tail of the scorpion, was effective against its bite; coleworts, which shun the vine, were a cure for drunkenness; and cyclamen, with its ear shaped leaves, was a cure for deafness.

Another key aspect to this magical approach was the concept that the greater attracted the smaller. This led to a heroic cure for bad breath which was proposed by Sir Kenelm Digby, a founder member of the Royal Society:

'Everyone knows, for example, that a greater stench will attract a lesser. It is an ordinary remedy, though a nasty one, that they who have ill breath hold their mouths open at the mouth of the privy, as long as they can, and by the reiteration of this remedy, they find themselves cured at last, the greater stink of the privy drawing unto it and carrying away the lesser, which is that of the mouth.'

Some of these concepts are not dissimilar to the ones which are regarded as the basis of homeopathy. Samuel Hahnemann originated homeopathy based on the principle that the hair of the dog that bites you is beneficial. His argument was that if a chemical agent produced the symptoms of the disease then the same agent given in minute quantities can cure it. The dilution of the medicine is crucial to its effectiveness, but the solution can be so dilute that the chances of finding one molecule of the original chemical still present is slim. This has led to the hypothesis that the fluid retains some memory of the molecule which influences the course of illness.

Many of these theories may seem bizarre to present-day doctors trained in scientific methods, but some practitioners of alternative medicine base their work on such concepts. It is always possible that future generations will look back at the scientific era with similar scepticism and amusement, but the notable successes of science, which are not confined to the medical field, hold out hope that the basic scientific philosophy is a solid foundation on which future progress can be built. The nature of this philosophy is discussed in the next chapter.

Empirical Medicine

As well as the practical surgical approach to medical problems, there is also an empirical side to physicians' skills. The Brahmian period of Indian medicine saw not only the development of surgical techniques but also the introduction of the five active procedures, namely emetics, purgatives, water enemas, oil enema and sneezing powder, as well as the utilization of hygiene and diet. China had its materia medica which introduced rhubarb, iron, castor oil, ginseng (which has a diuretic effect), and rauwolfia subsequently used as an anti-hypertensive in the form of reserpine. Egyptians had 876 remedies at their disposal with over 500 different substances, a therapeutic decadence which cried out for the introduction of a prescription policy! Arabian medicine is best remembered for its extensive pharmacopoeia, their expertise in chemistry and the preparation of medicine originating from their interest in alchemy. Many drugs used in modern medicine owe their origin to the empirical use of herbal remedies, and there can be no better example of this than Withering's discovery of the beneficial effect of foxglove in heart failure.

The discovery of America led to a significant exchange not only of diseases such as smallpox and measles to the New World and syphilis to the Old, but also of herbal remedies. By the end of the 18th century one third of the European pharmacopoeia had originated in America. Cinchona bark—containing quinine—from Peru was widely used for fever and it is thought that malaria was widespread in Europe at the time. Ipecac for diarrhoea, guaiacum for syphilis, and sarsaparilla as a diuretic are just some of the medicines imported.

Observation and Classification

Accurate observation, which forms the foundation of the modern scientific approach to medicine, can be traced back to Hippocrates (5th century BC) who was widely regarded as the father of medicine. What was particularly remarkable about Hippocrates was the combination of accurate description and practical management of disease with the laying down of ethical rules which are still the basis for medical practice today. All doctors would do well to heed his advice to first do no harm to your patient. It has even been suggested that a plaque be prominently displayed in hospitals stating that, 'There are some patients we cannot help, but no patients we cannot harm.' His first aphorism, 'Life is short and the art long; opportunity fleeting, experiment dangerous and judgement difficult', is particularly relevant for a book on uncertainty.

Galen (130–200) was strongly influenced by Hippocrates to whom he acknowledged his debt. In time, Galen's authority was such that his ideas dominated medical teaching for centuries. Aureolus Theophrastus Bombastus von Hohenheim (1490–1541), more conveniently known as Paracelsus, was so infuriated by the continuing influence of Galen that he prefaced some of his lectures by burning any book of Galen that he could find which, no doubt, did not endear him to the local librarian. Paracelsus had a reputation for forthright opinions enthusiastically propounded, hence the term bombastic which is derived from his name. However, notwithstanding Paracelsus' strictures, Galen's reputation was well founded. He stressed the importance of accurate anatomical knowledge and contributed extensively to this by his dissection on apes and pigs. He could also be said to have founded experimental physiology with such experiments as tying the ureter to show that the kidney produced urine.

The practice of observation and accurate description of disease was largely subjugated to Galen's authority for several centuries until Thomas Sydenham's (1624–89) accurate and beautiful description of such diseases as gout. He was the first to distinguish clearly between scarlet fever and measles as well as chorea and hysteria.

In France, Pierre Bretanneau (1778–1862)—who developed the concept of specificity—was particularly influential. In many diseases he attributed a whole range of clinical and pathological features to a single cause, as with dothienenteritis which subsequently became known as typhoid. A disease was thus seen as a specific entity with widely different symptoms and signs resulting from a common cause.

The classification of disease based on observation was an important step in the communication of knowledge, and some enthusiastic taxonomists, like Linnaeus (1624–89) and Sauvages (1706–67), even believed it was possible to distinguish between genera and species of disease along the lines which have been used so successfully for plants and animals. The empirical tradition in Britain may have been the reason why so many diseases were well described by British physicians in the 18th and 19th centuries: this was particularly notable in Dublin where Graves, Stokes, Cheyne, Adams and Corrigan worked, and Guy's Hospital with Addison, Bright and Hodgkin.

In the 18th century in Paris, Pinel, Cabanis and others were keen to apply the analysis of symptoms to the understanding of disease, but their analysis was limited because their rich patients were averse to having their bodies examined, alive or dead. The French Revolution changed all that, with physicians becoming more practical people willing to learn about disease from necropsy study. Bichat (1771–1802) performed many hundreds of necropsies and laid down the foundation for our understanding of disease in terms of pathological anatomy. He died at the age of 30 from a fever contracted from one of his corpses, having by that age written three seminal books which established him—in some eyes—as the Newton of medicine. Pathological anatomy became the key to diagnosis and this still dominates medical thinking today.

The development of large hospitals for the 'common people', following the French Revolution, allowed treatment to be tested objectively, there no longer being a need to satisfy the whim of private patients. Before this, even the great physicians such as Laennec, Pinel and Cabanis were notorious for their nihilistic attitude. In Britain, treatment was more active which led to a cynical comment that the English kill their patients whilst the French let them die.

Scientific Medicine

During the 19th century it became increasingly obvious that diseases could not be adequately described purely in terms of abnormal anatomy—function was also important. Although William Harvey (1578–1657) could be regarded as the father of modern physiology with the discovery of the circulation of the blood, it was Johannes Müller (1801–58) in Bonn and Claude Bernard (1813–78) in Paris who developed physiology as a distinct science, applied not only to disease in humans and animals, but also to normal biological function. Later, basic biological research led to discoveries such as insulin by Banting and Best which profoundly affected medical practice.

The foundation of pathophysiology was laid down by Virchow (1821–1902), one of Müller's students, with his work on thromboembolism and tumour growth. In the process he developed pathology as a discipline at the microscopic level leading to the birth of modern histopathology. His work emphasized the cell as the basis of physiology and pathology leading to a movement away from histology to cytology as the focus of progress.

As the successes of basic science accumulated, inevitably the study of disease drifted towards the laboratory and away from the patient. Whilst there were clear disadvantages in this, the rewards have been considerable. One of these has been the development of microbiology which has profoundly influenced our effectiveness in treating many diseases.

The contagious nature of many diseases was recognized before microbiological agents were discovered. The treatment of lepers, for example, was unbelievably callous because of their infectivity; in many cultures they were declared legally dead and hounded from society. The heroic efforts of the inhabitants of Eyam in Derbyshire to limit the spread of Black Death by isolating the whole village would not have been made unless they knew that the illness was contagious. Even the relationship of putrefaction and ill health was known to Rhazes (850–923), the first of the Arabian doctors to achieve worldwide fame. When asked to decide the location of a new hospital in Baghdad, he hung pieces of meat at various points in the city and advised that the hospital be built where the putrefaction was slowest.

By the time that Semmelweiss (1818–65) had conclusively demonstrated the infective nature of puerperal fever, and John Snow (1813–85) had dramatically proved that cholera was spread by contaminated water, the contagious nature of many diseases was recognized, but the nature of the infective agent was unknown, despite use having been made of this knowledge through the development of inoculation and vaccination. Inoculation with small amounts of smallpox had been used in China and Turkey before being described in the USA by Zabdiel Boylston (1679–1766). Not only did he inoculate his two black slaves, which was probably considered an acceptable risk at that time, he also inoculated his own son. Furthermore, in the finest experimental tradition, he exposed them all to the disease in the local pesthouse without any ill effects!

This approach was made safer by Edward Jenner (1749–1823) who overheard a dairymaid's remarks to the effect that she could not get smallpox because she had already had cowpox. In 1796 he vaccinated his first patient with cowpox and, exceeding even Boylston in scientific zeal, he proved its effectiveness by safely injecting the patient with a good dose of smallpox.

By the middle of the 18th century the time was ripe for the birth of microbiology, and there is no disputing that the brilliant chemist, Louis Pasteur (1822–95), in a series of vital experiments, laid down the foundation of this discipline. He showed that fermentation was due to contamination with airborne organisms and he extended the concept to human illness. As well as taking the work of Jenner further, particularly with vaccination for rabies, he discovered stereochemistry and saved the French silk industry by discovering why silkworms were dying. There is little wonder that virtually every town in France has a Rue Pasteur. The work of Pasteur and Koch (1843–1910)—who did much to identify and classify many bacteria such as cholera, anthrax and tubercle bacillus—led to the introduction of effective treatment for infections after the discovery of arsphenamine by Ehrlich and penicillin by Fleming. Koch's postulates, describing the four steps required to confirm that a particular organism causes a particular disease, remain valid to this time.

Over the last century we have seen the emphasis put on the cause and pathogenesis of disease, with rational treatment directed accordingly. This can be seen in Ehrlich's successful search for the magic bullet which destroys bacteria without harming the patient. Important therapeutic advances have also been made through our understanding of physiology as in the development of beta blockers and H2 antagonists by Sir James Black. As well as being intellectually satisfying this approach has undoubtedly been very successful, but despite this there has been a reversion, beginning in British and American medicine, towards a greater emphasis on the empirical evaluation of treatment. It is unsatisfactory to accept the efficacy of treatment simply because it is logical and the question has to be asked, 'Does it work in practice?' This has led to the increasing application of statistics in medicine and the evolution of the controlled clinical trial. Gavaret foresaw this one hundred years earlier in his remarkable book *Principes Généraux de Statistique Médicale* in which he laid down ten tenets which form the basis of the medical statistical approach.

This century has seen an explosion in our knowledge of disease through improved understanding of physiology and immunology leading to effective treatment in all branches of medicine. This has occurred alongside rapid advances in anaesthesia and surgery leading to transplant surgery, artificial joints and in vitro fertilization. More recently we have witnessed considerable progress in our understanding of the genetic basis of disease which holds promise for the future effective prevention and management of inherited disease. There have also been major advances in the diagnosis of disease through such technical innovations as fibre-optic endoscopy, computer tomography and nuclear magnetic resonance. Modern medical practice becomes so successful that a new set of problems has become increasingly relevant, namely problems associated with ageing and difficulties in adequate funding of health care services.

Conclusion

This brief review is intended to highlight the major directions that medical practice has taken since civilization began, with a view to understanding what we mean by the term disease. Undoubtedly the classification and accurate description of human ailments into categories called diseases was an important step in our understanding of illness, encouraging communication of knowledge and ideas. Initially diseases were defined as a cluster of clinical features called syndromes, like rheumatic fever, and many of these syndromes still retain the eponymous names of the physicians who first described them accurately, such as Reiter's and von Recklinghausen's disease. Occasionally, the disease was named solely on the basis of a symptom, myasthenia gravis for example, or a sign such as erythema nodosum.

The gradual evolution of the scientific method, and its application to medicine, has revolutionized medical practice by revealing the cause of many illnesses. This process of discovery has often been in steps, with the morphological basis of disease being defined first. This has led to many diseases being named according to the pathological anatomy, for example nephritis and hepatic cirrhosis. In some cases this is as far as our knowledge of disease has progressed. In other cases the cause of disease is better understood. Many diseases are not even associated with a clearly abnormal anatomy, but can be defined in physiological (atrial flutter), biochemical (porphyria) or microbiological (amoebiosis) terms. Because our understanding of the various medical conditions is at different stages, some diseases are still classified according to a set of clinical features whilst others are classified in terms of pathology or aetiology. Is there little wonder that the term disease causes confusion?

DISEASE—A SUGGESTED DEFINITION

Many people think of a disease as an agent which causes illness. Problems caused by infection lend some credence to this view because an identifiable agent, the micro-organism, can be isolated. Undoubtedly we do 'catch' infections, but classifying disease in terms of these infectious agents is unsatisfactory because the same agent can produce very different illnesses. Infection with haemolytic *Streptococcus*, for example, can produce diseases as different as erysipelas and puerperal fever, and Epstein–Barr virus is implicated in diseases as varied as Burkitt's lymphoma, glandular fever and nasopharyngeal carcinoma.

Is it possible to define disease in aetiological terms even if we abandon any hope of describing disease purely in terms of an external cause such as an infectious agent? This already looks unlikely from the examples just given, and there are many other examples of pathological processes which can produce widely different diseases. Atheroma, for instance, can produce diseases as different as myocardial infarction, cerebrovascular accident and intermittent claudication. Even if our knowledge of aetiology was complete the classification of disease in terms of cause can never be satisfactory. Abnormalities of structure and function, the basis of symptoms and signs, must be taken into account when disease is classified yet these too cannot provide a satisfactory taxonomy alone. Most bacterial pneumonias look very much alike when the lung is examined down a microscope, and the clinical features are similar, but the nature of the infecting organism is crucially important in the management of the patient. Diseases have to be described in terms of aetiology as well as in the pathology or pathophysiology which results. Considering diseases solely as causes of illness is simply not tenable.

Since disease cannot be regarded as really existing independently of the ill person, a nominalist approach to the definition of disease is likely to be more promising. As Campbell et al. (1979) point out,[3] a definition should answer the question, 'What do you mean when you use the name of a disease?' rather than, 'What is a disease?' The definition of disease provided by Scadding[5] uses this approach; despite its limitations it may be as near as we are likely to get to a satisfactory working definition.

> 'The name of a disease refers to the sum of the abnormal phenomena displayed by a group of living organisms in association with a specified common characteristic or set of characteristics by which they differ from the norm for the species in such a way as to place them at a biological disadvantage.'

The study by Campbell et al.[3] shows that this definition is not appropriate to colloquial discourse when (a) the cause is an event or physical agent obvious to the patient or (b) the medical profession is not important in the diagnosis and treatment. But this is just a question of general usage; there is no reason why the above definition should not be applied to conditions such as carbon monoxide poisoning, fractured skulls or malnutrition.

Scadding's definition is not, however, without problems which are useful to explore if only to emphasize the difficulties in providing a comprehensive definition. He defines disease in terms of a *specific set of features* which is *abnormal* and *disadvantageous*. Of these the term disadvantageous, the least contentious, will be considered first.

Disadvantageous

Everyone can accept that broken arms, appendicitis and brain tumours are disadvantageous. Even relatively minor problems such as hay fever, rosacea and pruritus ani have a nuisance value although the disadvantage may be minor and in some cases hardly significant. There are, though, a few illnesses which are advantageous in certain circumstances. For example, to have sickle cell trait in malaria infested countries is advantageous because of the resistance it provides against malaria. On the other hand, it is disadvantageous in hypoxic conditions when infarction may occur, and, in consequence, no one with sickle cell trait can hold a civil airline pilot's licence.

The interplay of illness and environment may also have led to the high prevalence of diabetes in American Indians conveying a survival value because of adaptation to food shortage. Similarly, mice susceptible to diabetes live much longer than normal mice when deprived of food. However, whilst there are some negative medical conditions with possible positive survival value, as in these examples, they are few and far between, so this aspect of Scadding's definition is the more readily accepted.

Abnormal

Abnormality, which is likely to be a key feature in any definition of disease, can be difficult to define. When a disease has a clear-cut clinical pattern such as myocardial infarction, there is unlikely to be any serious disagreement about abnormalities. Similarly, someone with thyrotoxicosis resulting in weight loss, tachycardia, tremor and exophthalmos can be readily recognized as being abnormal, but someone who has a marginally over-active thyroid leading to marginal weight loss perhaps associated with heightened alertness would be difficult to distinguish from some people with normal thyroid function and, in this case, there may even be some advantages to this abnormality.

The problem becomes particularly acute when considering diseases such as hypertension and obesity where there is considerable debate as to what is normal and abnormal. Risk factors increase in proportion to the blood pressure, but any dividing line between normal and abnormal can only be arbitrary. There are several problems in defining normality in these circumstances and one is particularly basic. In order to define a group as normal it is necessary to exclude abnormal people. But to exclude abnormal people it is necessary to know what is normal. The argument is therefore circular and the distinction between normal and abnormal arbitrary.

The choice of the population from which normality is defined is also influential in deciding what is normal and abnormal. Few would deny that dental caries are abnormal, yet in Western society they are virtually universal. In that dental caries are usually regarded as abnormal, in this case abnormality is defined in relationship to an idealized norm. Dyschromic spirochaetosis, a spirochaetal disease with significant morbidity and mortality, is so common in a South American tribe that those without it are regarded as abnormal and excluded from marriage. Most people would accept that it is a disease, but in that society it is not regarded as being abnormal.

Environmental factors can also influence normality. Japanese people brought up in Japan are shorter than Americans, but when reared on an American diet they are significantly taller than their Japanese cousins. The problems of expressing 'normality' were addressed by clinical chemists during the 1970s, and it was determined that results should be compared to a reference population appropriate to the patient. This is well illustrated in the lipid field where differences in dietary habits lead to widely different blood cholesterol levels in different nationalities. On the other hand, normality could be some form of idealized norm based on our concept of what is good and healthy. In turn, this may depend upon our knowledge or thoughts on disease processes: for example, there is good evidence that a high cholesterol level is associated with atheroma, so we accept as normal the level in a society with a relatively low cholesterol as this fits in with what we know about the physiological processes involved in atheroma.

We have, therefore, the choice of an empirical norm which applies only to the population studied, or an idealized norm based on our concept of what it should be like to be healthy. In either case it should be appreciated that normality is arbitrary and prescriptive.

Specific Set of Features

An even more contentious issue in Scadding's definition is the degree of specificity of the features by which a disease is recognized. To what type of features are we referring? Clearly the symptoms and signs of a disease are often not specific enough to characterize it. It is usually not possible, for example, to distinguish between ulcerative colitis and Crohn's disease of the large bowel from the history and any abnormal sign that may be present. Similarly, the symptoms and signs of gout, due to deposition of uric acid in the joint, can be identical to the symptoms produced by deposition of calcium pyrophosphate.

When our knowledge of disease was scant there was little choice but to classify disease in terms of the readily observed features. However, as medical knowledge has increased over the last two centuries there has been an increasing trend to define disease in terms of abnormal anatomy and function. This reductionist approach has certainly proved to be useful but inevitably it leads to loss of information. Each patient is an individual who will respond in a unique way to a particular pathology. It is not enough to know that a patient has a duodenal ulcer; what really matters is the type of problem the ulcer is causing, if any. The presence of pathology may not be relevant, as when a gall stone is found in an elderly patient, or when the uric acid is raised in a patient with joint pain. However, the alternative approach of basing a diagnosis on the taxonomy of clinical features would be undeniably complex. The current aim of investigation is to make a diagnosis based on pathology, even if this is done by inference rather than direct examination. The popularity of the clinico-pathological conference—which takes the form of a clinical 'who dunnit' shortly to be solved by the pathologist—attests to this.

A satisfactory definition of disease would have to take into account all the features of a disease including the symptoms, signs, pathophysiology and aetiology. One practical problem in achieving this is that our knowledge of disease is incomplete. A further difficulty arises from the practical problems of sampling bias which influences our medical knowledge. These take two main forms:

1. Most research is undertaken in patients attending hospital and they often have more severe illness. Too often general statements are made about the management of disease based on research work performed on a selected group of patients. The severity of disease varies and a treatment that might be appropriate for the more severe case may not be appropriate for the less severe problems seen in general practice.
2. Much of our medical knowledge is based on cases which come to post mortem. Unless the pathological features of disease can be determined from specimens taken from the living patient they will only reflect the end stage of disease. Many classical textbook descriptions of diseases are based more on the pathological findings as found at post mortem than on the clinical disease usually seen. Rheumatic fever is now becoming a rare condition, but when rife it was uncommon to see it with the clinical carditis classically described.

A further complication in defining disease in terms of a specific set of features is that disease patterns change with time and place for varying reasons. Syphilis had a much more fulminating course in the Middle Ages and measles can be devastating in a community not previously exposed. This is true not only of infective illnesses—when the difference can be understood in terms of immunity—but also applies to some non-infectious diseases. Peptic ulceration has changed quite dramatically over the last century. Jennings[6] described in 1940 how country practitioners saw perforated ulcers commonly in young women which, 'Swept away beautiful and healthy creatures within a few hours.' Similarly, With[7] in Denmark in 1881 wrote about the common problem of haematemesis and performation from gastric ulcers in young women. Duodenal ulcer was rare, at least in those coming to post mortem. Duodenal ulcer has now become more common particularly in men, and there is a growing incidence of peptic ulcer in elderly people attributable to the use of non-steroidal anti-inflammatory drugs.

Treatment has also changed the presentation of disease. Most textbooks still describe features of disease which are now rarely seen. The frequent use of antibiotics by general practitioners has made the classical presentation of lobar pneumonia uncommon, and a patient with subacute bacterial endocarditis exhibiting Osler's nodes and Janeway lesions would be a rarity indeed. Common usage of cimetidine and similar drugs for the symptoms of peptic ulcer is making gastric perforation increasingly infrequent. Not that this necessarily changes the spectrum of disease, but it does influence the type of cases commonly seen.

These difficulties in defining disease cannot easily be overcome making it unlikely that there will ever be a durable classification of disease. Reznek[4] argues that there is no underlying order of disease awaiting discovery, and that inevitably the classification of disease must be arbitrary and imposed. Diseases do not have highly specific clusters of properties which distinguish one set of patients from another. That is, they do not fall into what the philosopher would call natural kinds. The classification in use has been arrived at for convenience and will inevitably change with increasing knowledge. Patients do not 'catch' diseases, they become ill and doctors impose a diagnosis on them for convenience. There is nothing wrong in doing this. It may be necessary for the practical management of individual patients, as well as for the ease of communication between doctors and also with their patients. Doctors should not be surprised, though, when they see patients whose illness does not easily fit into any recognized disease pattern. The designation of the patient as having a 'forme fruste' of a particular disease evades the issue but is often convenient for practical management.

This difficulty in defining the very thing that we spend much of our time trying to diagnose and treat is a fundamental problem in medical practice. Although it does not prevent us managing most medical problems satisfactorily, it does suggest that we should not get hooked on the need for a precise diagnosis in every case.

FURTHER READING

Camp, J. *The Healer's Art (The Doctor Through History)*. London: F. Muller, 1978.

Feinstein, A. R. *Clinical Judgement*. Baltimore: William and Wilkins, 1967.

Goldberg, A. Towards European Medicine: an historical perspective. *Journal of the Royal College of Physicians* 1989; **23**: 277–286.

King, L. S. What is disease. *Philosophy of Science* 1954; **21**: 193–203.

Reznek, L. *The Nature of Disease*. London: Routledge & Kegan Paul, 1987.

Singer, C. and Ashworth, E. *A Short History of Medicine*. Oxford: Oxford University Press, 1962.

2
Philosophy, Science and Medicine

'Medicine is a science of uncertainty and an art of probability.'

Osler

INTRODUCTION

With medical knowledge expanding remorselessly, it is hardly surprising that philosophy gets little or no attention in the medical syllabus. One can sympathize with the student who felt that the only further addition to the medical curriculum should be spare time, but a failure to question basic assumptions ultimately leads to stagnation. A discussion of ethical and social issues arising from the successful application of the scientific method is outside the scope of this book, but a basic understanding of the philosophical foundation of the scientific method is very relevant to an understanding of uncertainty as it applies to medical practice. In this chapter, the logical processes which underpin scientific philosophy will be discussed, from the hope that inductive or deductive logic would eventually lead to a comprehensive description of the physical world to the more realistic acceptance of the transient nature of scientific theories.

It is now accepted that scientific progress does not depend solely on the slavish collection of facts as implied with the inductive approach, nor is progress limited to the application of logical deductive thought. Both these are important, but it is the generation of hypotheses which is the real key to success. Some people have regarded this as an unscientific act, but it is a fundamental part of the scientific process. Whilst the generation of hypotheses may be based on established fact, it goes beyond what is known in a non-rational way. It is an intuitive leap into the unknown or, as Peter Medawar called it, a 'happy guess'.

However, a hypothesis without some attempt to justify it is of no lasting importance; its value lies in the predictions which can be made from it—these can be tested and a failure to confirm expectations leads to rejection of the hypothesis. This process of hypothesis generation, prediction and testing has been called the hypothetico-deductive method. It is important not only as the method of science, but also to the way we think in everyday life. The limitations of inductive and deductive logic, and their relationship to the hypothetico-deductive method, are explained in this chapter. An appreciation of the method can help in the day-to-day management of patients as illustrated by the use of this method in tackling difficult diagnostic problems. This is explored further in Chapter 3.

The concept of cause and effect, which arises from inductive logic, has been of great importance to science and also seems relevant to everyday thinking. Because of its importance, it is considered separately in this chapter. It is such a powerful concept that the Victorian scientist hoped that science would describe an orderly and predictable world and thought they were near to achieving that. The practical usefulness of science resides in the power it has of making reliable predictions, so the concept of cause and effect is attractive. Although enormous advances were made in the 18th and 19th centuries using such concepts, the limitations of this approach have become apparent in this century.

It was the search for a better understanding of subatomic particles and the forces that influence them which revealed a very basic problem in achieving a comprehensive understanding of our universe. Quite simply we cannot accurately know what is happening at this level without altering the very thing we are trying to measure. The influence of the observer is always a potential problem in making any measurement, but with larger masses and forces this effect can be made negligible. A lot of effort goes into experimental design to achieve this, although it is often not easy to realize in practice. However, the point is that at the subatomic level it is impossible even in theory to make accurate measurements and, therefore, impossible to make accurate predictions except on a statistical basis. The reason for this is stated in Heisenberg's principle of uncertainty which dominates quantum physics. Whilst these principles do not impinge on the daily life of a doctor it is salutary to consider them, because they demonstrate the fundamental uncertainty which lies at the heart of science.

There is a further situation in which simple rules of cause and effect do not operate and this is directly relevant to medical practice. Complex non-linear systems, as found in thermodynamics and weather patterns, do not behave predictably. For this reason scientific understanding of them has lagged behind that of relatively simple linear systems dealt with in Newtonian physics. The problems lie in defining the exact state of all the forces and matter involved in complex systems combined with the magnification of any error brought out by non-linear behaviour. The properties of such systems are now better understood and form the basis of the aptly named chaos theory. Biological systems are notoriously complex particularly when studied in their entirety. For this reason it is common to take a reductionist approach and study a relatively small aspect of physiology or biochemistry to allow control of the extraneous factors. However, the response of a patient to disease does not allow closely controlled experiments; the hope for a better understanding of medical outcomes in the future may reside in the application of chaos theory to medical problems.

It is impossible in this book to give more than a brief taste of these ideas which will be new to many doctors, but their role in limiting the certainty which we can hope to achieve is relevant to medicine. These limitations are built into the scientific foundation of medical practice.

THE HYPOTHETICO-DEDUCTIVE METHOD IN SCIENCE AND PHILOSOPHY

The way the human mind thinks is unlikely to have changed significantly in the history of civilization, but our understanding of the process has advanced considerably. Two philosophers in the early 17th century developed contrasting ideas on the thinking process, one with the rational and the other with the empirical approach. The method of logic is attributed to Descartes (1596–1650) and the method of experiment to Francis Bacon (1561–1626). As Bronowski[8] pointed out, the two men form an interesting contrast between what are usually held to be the French and British habits of thought. Descartes did most of his work in bed and Bacon is reputed to have died of a cold which he caught when he tried the experiment of stuffing a chicken with snow.

Inductive Logic

Although the ideas of inductive logic predated Bacon it is his name which is usually associated with this empirical approach to knowledge. The inductive approach stresses the importance of the unbiased observation collected without any preconceived notions. It is a particularly English philosophical tradition; John Locke (1632–1704), for instance, held that all knowledge could only be derived from sense experience. He viewed the mind as being like a blank paper onto which ideas are sketched through sensations. His friendship with Sydenham (1624–89) may well have influenced the latter's practical approach to medicine, based on observation and classification, which was an important step in the history of medicine.

Only when sufficient facts are collected can the inductivist seek principles or laws to explain them. He is allowed to widen his observations by tampering with experience in the form of an experiment, and this was encouraged by Bacon, but he should not speculate about possible principles before the evidence is collected in order to avoid the observation influencing the data. From particular observations he derives general principles which can then be used for making future predictions.

John Stuart Mill (1806–73), another Englishman, took the concept of inductive logic further by adding rules for reasoning. These rules of inductive reasoning were summarized in five canons, of which two were particularly powerful. His canon of agreement states that when two or more instances of a phenomenon have only one circumstance in common, that circumstance is the cause of the phenomenon. The canon of difference states that if an instance in which the phenomenon occurs and an instance in which it does not occur have every circumstance in common save one, that circumstance is the cause of the phenomenon. His concept of the scientific method thus centred around the importance of discovering causes. If the use of an antibiotic is associated with the cure of an infection in a way consistent with these two canons, it is said that the antibiotic is the cause of the cure. This has proved to be such a powerful idea that it is incorporated into common sense thinking, but it is not without problems, some of which are explored later in this chapter.

The inductivist approach, based on observation and collection of data, is familiar to all students of medical science. The knowledge that the pain of arthritis, for example, can be improved by taking non-steroidal anti-inflammatory drugs is well established and based on observation. This would seem to be a simple example of the inductive process at work, but there are several important questions that could be raised concerning the type, amount and quality of data obtained.

Why, for instance, should a drug belonging to this class have been given to people with arthritis in the first place, unless the speculation is that the pain might be relieved? It is, of course, possible that people with arthritis would have been given the drug accidentally and the observation made that the pain was relieved. The finding that foxglove cured dropsy was presumably made in this way. However, scientific progress would have been tediously slow if advances had to wait on such fortuitous observations. Even when fate is kind to the research worker, as when a penicillin mould contaminated Fleming's culture plate, the opportunity for a scientific breakthrough could be missed unless the scientist has some idea about what to look for. Fleming could easily have discarded his culture plates if he had not been looking for a substance which could destroy bacteria.

The truth is that the idea of the unbiased observation is a myth. No one really believes that the mind is a clean slate on which the records of the sensations are inscribed. Sense data are chosen, simplified, and interpreted before being committed to memory. One of the weaknesses of the inductive method is that there is no incentive written into it to guide one in the choice of observations to make. As Peter Medawar[1] put it. 'We cannot browse over the field of nature like cows at pasture.' In doing so we might stumble upon an observation which has fundamental implications, but as likely as not we would not recognize its importance unless it fitted some theory or idea we already had in mind.

A further weakness of the inductive approach arises from the question as to how much data should be collected before a general statement can be made. An imprecise answer would be the more the better. The knowledge that the sun has come up every day in recorded history makes it a reasonably safe bet that it will rise tomorrow. This is not, however, a perfectly safe assumption. Bertrand Russell[9] put it wryly: 'The man who has fed the chicken every day throughout its life at last wrings its neck instead, showing that more refined views as to the uniformity of nature would have been useful to the chicken.' The discovery that six people with asthma improved with desensitization to allergens would not be a good foundation on which to introduce this potentially dangerous practice. It often is difficult with complex systems to derive a clear principle or law which would apply without exceptions to future events, and one can then only summarize the findings in statistical terms.

However much information is collected, any generalization from it must go beyond the limits imposed by these observations. It was the Scottish philosopher David Hume (1711–76) who first pointed out this basic flaw in inductive logic. Any generalization allowing predictions about an infinite number of possibilities from a finite number of observations is unsound. Above all it is this leap beyond the observations which is the fatal weakness in inductive logic.

Deductive Logic

The alternative type of reasoning, described and developed by Descartes, is that of deductive logic. It differs fundamentally from inductive logic by arguing from the general to the particular. The starting point is a number of self-evident axioms which apply to all circumstances. Using a set of infallible principles of inference it is possible to derive specific consequences which are bound to be right assuming, of course, that the axioms and principles of inference are correct in the first place. By using this method,

Descartes tried to do for philosophy what Euclid had done for mathematics, that is to build up a series of indisputable theorems from a series of basic axioms.

There are now several systems of logic which can be used in the inference process, but the system of Aristotle (384–322 BC) based on syllogisms will suffice to demonstrate the principle. Aristotle's influence on the theory of logic was so profound that it held sway for 2000 years until the modern revival of this branch of philosophy. The advantage of using these old fashioned syllogisms is that, unlike the propositional calculus now widely used in logical argument, they do not require familiarity with a symbolic notation. What must be the most commonly quoted one is:

All men are mortal.   (premise)
Socrates is a man.   (premise)
Therefore: Socrates is mortal.   (conclusion)

Any form of deductive logic is open to potential criticism both on the basis of the axioms chosen and the inference used. Take the above example for instance. All men are mortal is a statement based on a limited number of observations and, whilst it is a fairly safe generalization, it is possible in future that some men will be immortal. Axioms based on observations in this way are vulnerable to the same argument used by Hume so devastatingly for inductive logic.

On the other hand, axioms based on irrefutable truths are more limiting. Descartes considered that 'all things that we conceive very clearly and very distinctly are true' should be the basis of believing a statement to be axiomatic. His ultimate basic premise 'I think therefore I am' is widely known, but other premises are more contentious. Any system of knowledge based on axioms depends ultimately on the soundness of these initial assumptions. If they are uncontentious the tendency is for them to permit no more than the deduction of trivia. In the development of complex deductive systems the initial stages often look promising, but before long the system becomes complex and unwieldy with an ever increasing need for further implausible assumptions. It is no surprise that, as with Carnap (1891–1970) and Leibniz (1646–1717), the programme was started but never completed.

Even Aristotle admitted to the problem of defining the basic universal premises and tried to establish these premises 'on the evidence of groups of particulars which offer no exception'. This implies observation followed by generalization, an empirical approach which is primarily inductive, despite the Greek tradition of holding practical matters in contempt.

Acceptance of basic axioms, therefore, can be contentious whether they are based on observation or seem to be obviously true. There are also potential problems in the process of inference. The inferences used in deductive logic are derived from a number of self-evident principles. Three of these have been singled out by tradition under the name of 'laws of thought':

1. The law of identity: 'Whatever is, is.'
2. The law of contradiction: 'Nothing can both be and not be.'
3. The law of excluded middle: 'Everything must either be or not be.'

Such principles are regarded as 'known to us' not through experience but innately. This implies being born with this knowledge and for this reason many prefer to use the term 'a priori'. Lengthy discussion on the difficulties in logical inference would not be appropriate in this book, but a simple example will demonstrate the sort of difficulties that can arise when too simplistic a view of logic is taken, even with straightforward syllogisms. Take, for example, the argument:

All Britons are European.
All Welsh are European.
Therefore, all Welsh are Britons.

This takes the form:

All As are Cs.
All Bs are Cs.
Therefore, all Bs are As.

Although this may seem sensible at first sight, the inference as it stands is invalid. Substituting Germans for Welsh makes this immediately apparent.

Despite being powerful logical systems, both inductive and deductive logic have serious flaws. Their main value may be in justifying conclusions which have been arrived at by using more intuitive processes. Stuart Mill eventually acknowledged this possibility for inductive logic when he concluded that even if his reasoning was not a true method of discovery at least it was the sole method of proof. In deductive logic it is recognized that there is both a synthetic and an analytical approach. The first starts with first principles not based on observation—a priori premises—from which conclusions can be drawn. This is a logically consistent approach but suffers from the limitations mentioned above, namely the difficulty in identifying sufficient uncontentious axioms to allow development of a comprehensive understanding of the world. The analytical thinker, on the other hand, begins with the proposal he wishes to prove and tries to trace its origin back to first principles. This Descartes defended with the argument that the basic axioms are not likely to be accepted by all. In saying this Descartes was inconsistent in his method; although supposedly synthetic it was, in fact, often analytical.

Despite the problems of inductive logic outlined in this chapter, there can be no doubt that the empirical approach to medicine has been of key importance in the development of modern medical practice. The more deductive approach, arguing from basic premises such as the existence of four humours, ultimately led nowhere. However, an approach based on blind observations leads to slow progress although this may well have been the way an early pharmacopoeia was developed. What is needed is some guiding light to point to the observations which need to be made. This is provided by the generation of hypotheses.

The Role of Hypotheses

The importance of a hypothesis is that it provides a reason for collecting specific data with the aim of testing that particular theory. Without this the process becomes haphazard and inefficient. This idea had occurred to many people before William Whewell's (1974–1866) cogent arguments led to the acceptance of its central importance in the thinking process. Some, possibly influenced by the rigours of the inductive process, rejected hypotheses as being unscientific. Newton (1642–1727), for example, claims to have 'feigned no hypothesis' and Thomas Reid (1710–1796) of the 'Scottish school of common sense' considered that hypotheses should be treated with contempt. In his book *The Philosophy of the Inductive Sciences* Whewell[10] considered the role played by observation and experimentation in the advance of science (incidentally, it was Whewell who first coined the term scientist). He pointed out that scientific discoveries proceeded not by blind collection of observations, but by collecting facts guided by a conceptual framework. Athough it is difficult to perceive of a hypothesis being generated out of the blue without reference to some observations which it is intended to explain, he emphasized that a hypothesis is generated at an early stage in the process of logical thought.

The formation of a hypothesis is not in itself a logical process and perhaps for this reason many consider it to be an art rather than the central pivot of science. Peter Medawar[1] claimed that people often confused the issue when they talked about the art of medicine. 'It is the unbiased observation, the apparatus, the ritual of fact finding and the inductive mumbo-jumbo that the clinician thinks of as scientific and the other element, intuitive and logically unscripted which he thinks of as creative art.' There is truly a marriage between the two, but Medawar considered that doctors were apt to get the bride and groom confused. The generation of a hypothesis, although intuitive, is at the heart of the scientific method.

The first step in the scientific process is, therefore, the generation of a hypothesis. This does not, however, lead to significant advances without the next step—the testing of hypotheses.

The Testing of Hypotheses

The strength of a hypothesis is not that it explains the observations already known, although this is clearly important, but that it can be used to make predictions which can then be tested. This predictive process uses deductive logic, and the combination of this with the generation of hypotheses is known as the hypothetico-deductive method. However, there is little point in developing a hypothesis which cannot be tested. The Vienna school of logical positivists, in their famous verifiability principle, considered a hypothesis to be worthless unless it could be put to a practical test and verified. They regarded many philosophical questions such as, 'Is there a God?', as being meaningless. A medical example of a meaningless statement is, 'It is morally wrong not to tell patients the truth about their diagnosis.' You can have strong beliefs about the right or wrong of this, but to attempt to prove it would be a fruitless exercise. On the other hand the statement, 'This person has a fractured femur', is meaningful because it can be tested.

However, as C. S. Pierce (1839–1914), one of the American pragmatist philosophers, pointed out, a scientific hypothesis can be fallible even when seemingly verified. An example of this was provided by Paracelsus who was supposed to have developed a sympathetic powder which could heal at a distance. When this salve was smeared on the weapon which had caused the wound the virtues present in this preparation were attracted to the wound by a sort of magnetic sympathy. Patients treated in this way seemed to fare better than those who had their wounds dressed repeatedly by the contaminated hands of physicians so appearing to confirm the hypothesis. Since most wounds heal when left to themselves this was not surprising, and we would no longer accept the original hypothesis, preferring to interpret the findings in terms of modern germ theory.

This type of problem led Karl Popper (1902–) to reason that you cannot prove any hypothesis. Whilst an observation may be consistent with a theory, you cannot generalize by saying that all observations will be consistent with this theory. This jump is similar to that taken in inductive logic which Hume criticized. You can, however, falsify a hypothesis. For example, the universal statement, 'All swans are white', cannot be proved; even if all swans seen have been white, the next one might be black. On the other hand, the converse statement, 'No non-white swans will be found', can be disproved and was so when black swans were found in Australia.

Popper argued, therefore, that a good hypothesis is one that is readily falsifiable. A hypothesis that cannot be tested and falsified is of little or no value. In the course of time a hypothesis that has survived several attempts to disprove it may be honoured with the title of theory or law, but even the strongest of theories may be eventually falsified. A classic example of this was when the physics developed by Einstein replaced the highly useful, but fundamentally flawed, physics of Newton.

As Popper pointed out, science does not rest on solid bedrock. The theories of science may account for many observations and work in practice, but as more penetrating observations are made their inadequacies will become apparent. New theories will replace old theories to give a more comprehensive explanation of nature, but we cannot expect to develop theories which will adequately explain all things for all time. The purpose of science is to describe the world in an orderly fashion and help us look ahead. It is not to develop absolute certainty, which is unobtainable.

The book *Logic of Scientific Discovery*, written by Karl Popper in 1959[11] is closely argued and has been enormously influential, although it cannot be recommended for light bedtime reading. Nevertheless, there are problems in the implementation of the concept of falsification of hypotheses. If there are, for example, two competing hypotheses, both consistent with the known observations, how does one decide which is nearer the truth? At the practical level this may not matter if both explain the observations adequately, and the competition will encourage the design of experiments to distinguish between them. However, this may not be possible with the technology of the time, and when faced with two theories both adequately explaining the facts there is a tradition to choose the simplest theory, applying what has been called Occam's razor. This gives a kind of aesthetic satisfaction but the philosophical justification for this is unclear; perhaps the simplest theory is the most general and therefore the most easily falsified. Darwin's theory of evolution provided a simple explanation of diverse observations which had previously led to multiple theories, many of them untestable.

Another problem with using falsification as a strict criterion for disproving and therefore eliminating a hypothesis is that it assumes the absolute accuracy of observation and interpretation. If an experiment is performed badly, for whatever reason, and the mistake is not obvious, a correct hypothesis could be eliminated prematurely and forgotten. This could have happened when an experiment on beta decay, a process by which a nucleus changes through emission of an electron or positron, was found to be inconsistent with the otherwise neat theory devised by Richard Feynman, but he wisely advised co-workers not to be down-hearted and to wait and see. A few days later an experimental error in the original work was reported and their theory vindicated.

There are many examples in the scientific literature where a hypothesis has not been consistent with all the observations, but has not been discarded. A classic example of this concerned the orbital path of Uranus. This was inconsistent with Newton's theories, but the observation did not lead to the rejection of these theories. Further observation led to the discovery of an hitherto unknown planet subsequently named Neptune which was distorting the orbital path of Uranus. An attractive hypothesis may, therefore, be maintained even when observations are not consistent with it. The problem may simply be that technology is not advanced enough to make the appropriate observations possible. Another example is the circulation of blood, as proposed by William Harvey, which was not consistent with the knowledge existing at the time. It needed the discovery of capillaries by Malphigi (1628–94) before the theory was substantiated.

A further weakness of the falsification approach is the difficulty of applying it to the situation where the outcome can only be predicted on a basis of probability. A theory may state that an observation should occur so rarely that the discovery of this would make the theory very unlikely. Nevertheless, the confirmation of the observation can never falsify the theory with absolute certainty. Because of the probabilistic nature of the theory there is always a chance that the observation might be made however unlikely that might be. Quite apart from this, the limited accuracy of measuring instruments ensures that many observations cannot be stated with a precision which allows definite confirmation of a hypothesis.

Despite these objections it is generally accepted that the strength of a good hypothesis is that it makes precise and testable predictions. Confirmation of these predictions is particularly rewarding when a hypothesis has unexpected implications. The idea that light bends when passing near a large mass such as a star, as predicted by Einstein, must have offended the common sense of most people. The confirmation of this by Eddington (1882–1944) during a total solar eclipse in 1919 was a particularly impressive confirmation of the general theory of relativity. This theory had been rigorously tested and could not be disproved.

The Scientific Paradigm

The philosophical arguments in favour of falsification as the sole means of testing a hypothesis are impressive, but the principle has certainly not been applied universally. The examples given above are just a few of many instances which could be quoted. Arguing from a study of the history of science, Thomas Kuhn[12] pointed out that research in any one period seems to be performed within a relatively rigid framework or paradigm, an example of which would be Newton's theories of motion. When a new way of looking at the world is first developed most experiments performed are directed at proving the predictions arising from the paradigm to be correct. As long as the paradigm is sound most experiments are consistent with expectations and the odd experiment not in agreement is regarded as insufficient evidence to disprove it. What tends to happen, however, is that in time the paradigm becomes exhausted; new findings become increasingly difficult to fit into it; and auxiliary theories developed to explain new findings often become less and less plausible.

Even at this stage, the paradigm will still have its practical uses, but it is unsuitable for further conceptual development. The time is ripe for a shift to a new framework of thinking: although initially this may explain little more than the old paradigm, it usually has more potential for development. An example of such a change on a grand scale is the transition from classical Newtonian physics to relativity theory.

The new paradigm may not, however, be accepted unless it can be tested using the technology prevailing at the time. Aristorchus in the 3rd century BC anticipated Copernicus (1473–1543), but our knowledge of planetary movement at the time of Aristorchus, and for many centuries afterwards, was consistent with the seemingly simpler concept of Ptolemy which put the Earth at the centre of the solar system. As with many other scientists Aristorchus was before his time.

Popper would argue that experiments designed merely to support a hypothesis arising from within a paradigm is not true science, but most research is not on a grand scale dealing with fundamental scientific principle. Most research, including medical research, makes no attempt to introduce new fundamental ideas, but simply makes use of the principles already accepted to delve a little deeper into our understanding of nature. Whether hypotheses are generated to be proved or disproved may, to the practical person, be irrelevant. An experiment may be designed with the aim of proving a hypothesis, but if the observations are contrary to the hypothesis it ends up being disproved. However, whether a hypothesis is proved or disproved this should not necessarily be taken as the last word on this subject. A hypothesis may be proved by one experiment only to be disproved by another, perhaps better, experiment. Alternatively, a hypothesis may be disproved by a badly designed and performed experiment which subsequent work shows to be inaccurate. It does not pay to be too didactic on the basis of a single experiment. Uncertainty is central to the scientific method.

The Hypothetico-deductive Method of Reasoning

Whether one believes the philosophically pure concept of falsification of hypotheses or accepts what the history of science tells us about the testing of ideas, the generation of hypotheses, deduction of consequences and testing of these consequences is a powerful method of science. It is also an approach used in everyday life as well as in the diagnostic reasoning of doctors. The use in medical practice is explored in Chapter 3, but meanwhile an example of everyday use may convince the reader that the hypothetico-deductive method is a plausible method of reasoning.

If your car fails to start in the morning, how would you or a garage mechanic set about tracing the fault? I would suggest that you would develop a number of possible hypotheses, of which the following are a few:

1. That there may be an electrical fault with no current to the spark plug.

2. That there may be a failure of fuel supply to the carburettor.
3. That the starter motor may have jammed.

Observations can then be made to distinguish between these possibilities. If the engine is turning over, then the starter motor is working, so eliminating the third hypothesis. The plugs could be taken out and checked for a spark as the engine is turned. If a spark is present then it is likely that the fuel supply is at fault. Several further hypotheses can then be generated as to why the fuel supply is at fault, not least of which would be that the fuel tank is empty, something which the wise motorist would have checked first! Even if the reader is more prone to give the car a good kick and phone up the garage than hypothesize in the morning, at least it may be accepted that the hypothetico-deductive approach is likely to provide a quicker answer than the inductive approach of checking tyre pressure, exhaust system and safety belts without thinking of likely causes of the fault.

CAUSALITY AND STATISTICAL TRUTH

Cause and Effect

Even though the philosophical analysis of cause remains unsatisfactory, the concept of cause and effect dominated scientific thinking for several centuries. Newton's world was that of a series of events causally connected, and it was the highly successful Newtonian physics that led to the Industrial Revolution with the improvement in the quality of life which followed. From the motions of planets to the behaviour of billiard balls, the method of causes and mechanisms operated to such an extent that Laplace (1749–1827) argued that the whereabouts and speed of all things could be forecast from now to eternity if only one knew the current position of every atom and the strength of its forces. This mechanistic world was so central to the thinking at the time that Lord Kelvin (1824–1907) would not accept any idea as scientific unless he could either visualize or construct a model of it, and the theory of evolution although well known to Darwin's grandfather, was not accepted until the cause, natural selection, was understood. The concept of cause seems fundamental to our way of thinking and this applies to medical practice. In the research field, the research worker aims to discover the cause of disease and in the clinical field the physician seeks the cause of illness.

So, what do we mean by cause and effect? Common sense tells us that it concerns associations between events and usually in time. If event B follows A it is said to be caused by A. In the simplest form this relationship is invariable; when a billiard ball is hit by a cue, the ball moves, and when a gas is heated in a sealed container the pressure increases. These effects are caused by a transfer of energy and the result of this transfer can be precisely calculated.

When the events are closely connected the concept of cause is easily applied; even when there are several steps involved as in $A \rightarrow B \rightarrow C \rightarrow D$ the cause or sequence may be well established and reliable. However, the situation is usually not so simple, and this is particularly true of biological systems. This was recognized in the empirical tradition by the use of terms such as necessary cause, sufficient cause, and causes which were both necessary and sufficient. To take a biological example: with pneumocystis pneumonia, infection with *Pneumocystis carinii* is necessary but not sufficient. Immuno-suppression is also necessary, but is also not sufficient. Both are required for the clinical illness of pneumocystis pneumonia. There are on the other hand other diseases where causative factors are both necessary and sufficient. An occluded coronary artery, would fall into this category as a cause of myocardial infarction.

However, the situation is not usually as straightforward as in these examples and, for that matter, the purists may argue that the above examples are not quite as unambiguous as they seem at first sight. An outcome often occurs as a result of a whole chain of events which are best regarded together as an effective causal complex. None of the various causes in the sequence may be essential even when, colloquially, they are regarded as the primary cause. A different set of causal factors could have the same end result and the choice of any one particular causal factor in this complex may be arbitrary.

Consider the patient with rheumatoid arthritis (RA) who takes non-steroidal anti-inflammatory drugs (NSAID) and has a peptic ulcer (PU). The ulcer leads to bleeding which causes iron deficiency anaemia. The causal sequence would be

$$RA \rightarrow NSAID \rightarrow PU \rightarrow Bleed \rightarrow \text{iron deficiency anaemia}$$

None of these causal factors are a necessary cause of iron deficiency anaemia, and all are potentially redundant since iron deficiency anaemia could, for example, be dietary. Only the bleeding is a sufficient cause of iron deficiency anaemia, but not everyone would regard this as the cause of the anaemia. People with different interests and axes to grind may regard non-steroidal anti-inflammatory drugs as the cause of the iron deficiency anaemia. It is also interesting that the disease may not be treated, at least in the first place, by rectifying the causal factors, but by increasing the dietary intake of iron in the form of iron tablets.

There are very few associations which have a simple and invariable causal pathway connecting them. Most events are connected by a series of possible causal pathways in parallel. Failure to appreciate this can lead to futile arguments about the cause of disease. Some people may argue that because 70% of cancers are caused by environmental factors, then 50% cannot be genetically determined. But these statements are quite compatible because, in many cases, both environmental and genetic factors influence disease.

The concept of causality is about association and the question arises as to whether cause and effect is simply the way the brain interprets associations or whether cause has any real separate existence. In the generative theory of causation, causality is regarded as a feature of the real world. Observations are necessary to see cause at work, but cause is a real mechanism however poorly it may be understood. On the other hand, the empirical view of causation is that cause and effect is no more than an invariable succession. When two events are invariably associated, the latter event is said to be caused by the earlier, but this may be no more than a limiting case of correlation. It has even been suggested that correlation can be no more than very highly probable, and when one event truly invariably follows another it may be no more than a tautology. One of the best known correlations in physics, that between the weight of a body and its inertia, is so perfect because, as shown in general relativity theory, gravitational fields and acceleration are simply different ways of looking at the same thing.

Causality vs. Probability

As mentioned in the introduction, science is about prediction; the aim is to predict the outcome when events interact. This is both to prove the soundness of the underlying concepts and to reap the practical benefits to individuals or mankind that might result. This could be achieved by breaking down associations into causative factors in the hope of being able to predict an outcome with accuracy. Alternatively, we could limit ourselves to relating events simply on an empirical, statistical, basis. In fact, these approaches are not mutually exclusive. When the relationship between events is complex it may be simpler and more practical to define this association in statistical terms, but this does not preclude a search for causative connections to improve accuracy of predictions. On the other hand, causal laws may owe their success to the fact that they are admirable approximations when the laws of chance combine to give overwhelming likelihood.

The problem with statistical statements is their lack of certainty when applied to the individual occasion. A sound statistical statement can be made concerning the correlation between two events—when the events in question have been studied long enough—and the relationship expressed as a frequential probability. Mathematical statistics is based on this type of probability, such as the frequency of heads when a coin is tossed. A sound statement can be made to the effect that when a coin is tossed 1000 times, it will come down heads approximately 500 times, and the limitation of this approximation can be stated precisely. What statistics cannot do is to tell you whether the coin will come down heads or tails next time it is tossed, and yet this is precisely the type of information usually required. It is in the hope of rectifying this uncertainty that we seek a chain of causation. The various factors influencing this chain can be measured and if the chain in question is comprehensive, the outcome can be predicted with certainty. At least that is the goal of this rational approach.

A medical example may help to clarify these contrasting approaches. Take an example of a patient presenting with jaundice. One approach to making a diagnosis would be to make a list of associations purely on a statistical basis. Previous experience may show that, in your practice, 50% of cases are due to hepatitis, 20% due to gall stones, 10% due to pancreatic carcinoma and so on. A long list of possible reasons for the jaundice can be drawn up and the probability of each stated. The next step would then be to search for clinical features to help confirm or refute the most likely diagnosis, and again this could be done on a statistical basis. Whilst this has attractions to the mathematically inclined, a practical difficulty usually encountered is that the probability of each diagnosis is not known. This provides the experienced physician with a major advantage in that she will have a better feel for the likelihood of a diagnosis even if she cannot state it explicitly. Further details of this way of looking at medical practice and its limitations are explored in Chapter 4.

An alternative to this expirical approach would be to think in pathological terms, with the causes of jaundice as being pre-hepatic, hepatic and post-hepatic. The physician would then use his basic knowledge of anatomy, physiology and pathology to search for features which would narrow down the range of possible diagnoses. If these features point to post-hepatic jaundice, the next step would be to think of the possible abnormalities which can cause blockage of the biliary tract such as stones, pancreatic carcinoma and inflammatory narrowing of the bile duct. This approach is essentially different from the statistical method; it is because of the difficulty in programming computers to generate hypotheses through this type of causal reasoning that computer aided diagnosis has been less successful than initially hoped for (see Chapter 5).

Limits to Causality

There are well known pitfalls in the approach of splitting correlations into a sequence of smaller steps of causation. One of the commonly quoted examples of this is the interpretation of the experiment in which the frog jumps when the experimenter shouts. When the legs are removed the frog no longer jumps in response, and the interpretation could be that the frog hears with its legs. There is no fault in this logic; we only see it as ridiculous because we have other knowledge available to us. But even a sensible sequence of causation may be seen to be wrong when more information becomes available. It is now regarded, although not universally accepted, that nitrates are useful in angina by off-loading the heart so reducing the work demand and, therefore, oxygen requirements. However, it is not unreasonable to argue, as it has been in the past, that the response to nitrates is due to coronary vasodilatation, the reduction in angina being due to the increased blood flow to the myocardium.

In considering causal connections care has to be taken not to confuse coincidence with cause. The finding that the density of television aerials in Dublin was strongly correlated with birth rate and infant mortality was an obvious example of an association not related to causality, except insofar as both are likely to be related to an increased density of population. In this case, some connection can be seen even though the findings are not directly related, but in many correlations no such relationship exists.

Apart from these practical considerations there are two fundamental limits to the concept of causality which have become apparent in this century. The first is the uncertainty principle which lies at the centre of quantum mechanics, and the second is the complex behaviour of non-linear systems of which biological organisms are prime examples. A clearer understanding of these non-linear systems has led to a theory of chaos where chaos and order exist side by side in a beautiful but bizarre world of strange attractors and fractal geometry.

Quantum theory shattered the apparently predictable world of 19th century science. The discovery that photons could sometimes behave like particles and at other times like waves gave the first inkling that all was not well with classical physics. This finding was particularly interesting since it seemed to throw new light on the old argument between Newton and Huygens (1629–95) as to the nature of light. Newton regarded light as being composed of small particles, whereas Huygens regarded it as a wave form. In a sense both were right.

Furthermore, electrons could behave even more unconventionally. Instead of keeping to a regular orbit around the atomic nucleus, like the planets orbit the sun, they suddenly move from one orbit to another seemingly instantaneously. In this process a quantum of energy was released or taken up. There is no obvious cause involved in this process; subatomic particles were no longer behaving like billiard balls. In fact, electrons are better considered as probability waves than as solid particles. The act of observation may fix the position or the momentum of a subatomic particle, but not both. This deficiency is embraced in Heisenberg's principle of uncertainty, a consequence of which is that every description of nature contains some irremovable doubt. We can never predict the future of a particle with complete certainty, nor can we be certain of its present. Once we have uncertainty at this level then the future is essentially uncertain, however overwhelmingly probable it may be. Without this knowledge it is impossible to know whether cause and effect operates—the question becomes meaningless because it cannot be tested. We might as well postulate that the subatomic particles are passed around by fairies.

It is ironic that in splitting down the relationship between events into ever closer associations, with a view to increasing certainty, uncertainty reappears at the subatomic level. Because the concept of causality cannot be tested in these circumstances this does not mean that cause and effect does not really exist, it simply means that we have no means of knowing. At this level predictions have to be made on a statistical basis. Not that this uncertainty was readily accepted by all scientists; even Einstein, who had done so much to revolutionize physics, could not accept this doubt. As he put it, 'God does not play dice with the World'. Nevertheless quantum physics is now firmly established, leaving the whole fabric of matter based on uncertainty.

Yet even more worrying to those who crave an orderly world is the discovery that uncertainty extends even to what is usually regarded as the most exact discipline of science, namely mathematics. When the logical structure of mathematical systems was considered by Gödel, it became apparent that even in purely abstract systems of axioms, such as those of Euclid, questions arise which have no answers. It is possible to formulate theorems which canot be shown to be either true or false. Thus, uncertainty extends to the world of mathematical logic.

These uncertainties do not have any immediate impact on the daily practice of the doctor, but they do serve to emphasize the uncertainty which lies at the centre of modern science. In contrast, the second type of basic uncertainty is particularly relevant to medical practice because it involves complex non-linear systems—the type of system which a doctor deals with all the time. An understanding of these systems came initially from a study of thermodynamic principles which show that non-linear dynamic equations describing events removed from equilibrium lead to what has been called deterministic chaos. These equations demonstrate that small differences in the initial conditions can result in vastly different outcomes when the system is non-linear. Although an outcome can be determined accurately when the initial conditions are known precisely, the problem is that they never are. Even in a simple system of three atoms in an enclosed space, it has been shown that the paths of the atoms cannot be determined with certainty because the smallest error in stating the initial conditions changes the outcome. When you consider that the position and velocity of a particle have to be described numerically, and knowing that there are many more irrational than rational numbers, it follows that some approximation has to be made, for an irrational number extends to an infinite number of numerals. This alone makes the outcome unpredictable.

Physics and mathematics have traditionally dealt with linear systems because it is possible and relatively easy to make testable predictions, at least when concerned with physics at a larger scale than the subatomic. Many systems found in nature, however, are non-linear. Whenever enough energy is inserted into such a system it is likely to be destroyed unless some dissipative mechanism is also present. Living organisms have an energy input from food metabolism and loss of energy through heat and so have all the necessary ingredients for chaos. The environment with which they interact is also non-linear so it is hardly surprising that an understanding of population dynamics resulting from the predator–prey competition was one of the first systems to benefit from the application of chaos theory.

A study of weather systems by Lorenz was one of the major landmarks in the development of chaos theory. Major determinants of the weather—such as atmospheric pressure—keep within reasonable limits even though at any future time their position within that boundary is not predictable with a high degree of certainty. A line mapping out the movement in time of these interacting parameters never crosses the same path. Such a system is essentially unpredictable for practical purposes particularly when the starting conditions cannot be accurately defined, but this is not to say that they are totally chaotic. The weather changes within reasonable boundaries. It is generally warmer in summer and colder in winter, but what you cannot do is predict a white Christmas with any certainty, particularly when there are still a few days to go. Despite these constraining factors, it is possible for minor influences to have profound effects. It has even been said that the flap of a butterfly's wing in South America could lead to a thunderstorm in Europe.

A pattern of change which has these properties has been called a 'strange attractor'. The system will keep within the boundaries of this strange attractor unless an unusually strong force switches it to another coexisting attractor. The alternative may, for example, be something called a 'fixed point attractor' to which the system will always gravitate, rather like water to the plug hole in the bath. The possibility of coexisting attractors may be particularly relevant to medicine. Several diseases are self-limiting, the disturbing factor—the disease—being too weak to pull the system away from its usual attractor. However, a stronger disturbance may be large enough to cause a switch to a fixed point attractor where the final end-point is death unless a suitably strong force pushes it back.

The chaos resulting from this type of uncertainty is essentially different from stochastic chaos. The latter is purely random whereas the former is determined by rules of causality; it is at the practical level in defining initial conditions where order collapses. This plus the amplifying effect of the non-linearity leads to the collapse of predictability. In complex systems, accurate predictions applicable to an individual system, such as a particular patient, become the exception rather than the rule.

Chaos theory deals precisely with the sort of problem which encompasses the human condition in both the narrower and the wider sense. An understanding of physiological problems such as cardiac dysrhythmias and electrical waves in the brain has already benefited from its application. It could well be a useful way of exploring the complex interaction between disease and treatment with a view to defining the limits imposed on achieving a predictable response. The potential for applying the theory to physiological mechanisms, disease processes and epidemiological phenomena is enormous.

In this chapter our search for increasing knowledge and certainty within the scientific world has led us to the shaky foundations of matter and logic and to the chaos inherent in complex non-linear systems. The uncertainties arising from these ideas throw doubt on the value of the concept of causation. But despite its limitations, the idea of cause and effect has been and remains important to our understanding of the everyday world as seen at the practical level. The truth seems to be that without a belief in cause and effect, without knowing that something will happen predictably, any common sense attempt to understand the world would be frustrated and scientific progress would be in jeopardy. This certainly seems true of medical progress whereby the search for the cause of disease has been an essential process in the evolution of medical understanding. It is difficult to imagine how a scientific approach to disease could have been successful without a conceptual framework of anatomy, physiology and pathology in which the idea of cause did not play an essential role. Without this conceptual framework, held together by bonds of causality, the accumulation of further information would have been haphazard leading to a collection of unconnected facts. Some of these facts would, by chance, prove useful, but a directed search for relevant information is far more efficient and leads to a much faster evolution of medical knowledge. No doubt this will be true for a long time to come, but an understanding of the behaviour of complex systems may well become increasingly important in the future.

FURTHER READING

Beck, S. D. *The Simplicity of Science*. Penguin Books, 1962.

Bronowski, J. *The Common Sense of Science*. Penguin Books, 1951.

Coveney, P. and Highfield, R. *The Arrow of Time*. London: W. H. Allen, 1990.

Gjertsen, D. *Science and Philosophy: Past and Present*. London: Penguin Books, 1989.

Gleick, J. *Chaos*. London: W. Heinemann, 1988.

Kuhn, T. S. *The Structure of Scientific Revolutions*. Chicago: The University of Chicago Press, 1962.

Medawar, P. *Induction and Intuition in Scientific Thought*. London: Methuen, 1969.

Medawar, P. *The Limits of Science*. Oxford: Oxford University Press, 1985.

Richards, S. *Philosophy and Sociology of Science: An Introduction*. Oxford: Blackwell, 1983.

Wulff, H. R., Pederson, S. A. and Rosenberg, R. *Philosophy of Medicine: An Introduction*. Oxford: Blackwell, 1986.

3
Diagnostic Reasoning

'The physician who is attending a patient . . . has to know the cause
of the ailment before he can cure it.'

Mo-tze (5th–4th century BC)

INTRODUCTION

In the first chapter it was argued that the classification of medical
conditions into well defined categories called diseases was an
important step in our understanding of the various maladies
which have afflicted mankind. Without this classification it is
difficult to envisage the discovery of the mechanisms which cause
disease and which, in turn, form the basis of rational treatment.
However insecure our definition of disease may be, without some
framework on which to hang our knowledge, meaningful
communication between doctors would be impossible.

But does this mean that the labelling of patients into diagnostic
groups is an essential step in their management? Much has been
written about patient-orientated (management) as compared with
doctor-orientated (diagnostic) medicine, with the implication that
the former is undertaken in general practice and the latter in
hospital. The tacit assumption is that caring medicine differs from
scientific medicine and is superior to it.

This seems an unnecessary and somewhat false division which
manages to be disparaging to both family practitioners and
hospital doctors. Sir Douglas Black[13] included it as one of the
false antitheses in medicine, and considered the true antithesis
of caring medicine as not scientific medicine, but simply bad

medicine. Any experienced doctor would agree that full and exhaustive investigation of all patients entering a doctor's surgery would be inappropriate and impossibly expensive, but even with the simplest of problems a tentative diagnosis should be sought, even though this may not involve any investigation other than taking a history of the main complaint. No precise diagnosis may be made in a patient who complains of abdominal pain yet looks well and has no abdominal tenderness, but in giving a prescription for an antacid or laxative the doctor is committed to a probable diagnosis.

How far one travels down the diagnostic path depends upon many circumstances, but managing illness without a precise diagnosis is always risky. The cachectic old man who has smoked all his life may well have end-stage respiratory failure or lung cancer, the distinction not being crucial to management, but he could have tuberculosis or an empyema, and response to treatment could then be good. Rational treatment depends on a firm working diagnosis and so does assessment of prognosis. Inappropriate reassurance or unnecessary dissemination of gloom are penalties to be paid for taking too lax an approach to the diagnostic process. Both are unfortunate, although the latter may result in the benefit of a relieved patient who, with luck, may even attribute his good fortune to the efforts of his doctor.

For these good reasons, making a diagnosis becomes a major aim in hospital practice when missing a diagnosis can almost be regarded as a crime leading to feared condemnation from colleagues. As a result of this, there is a greater tendency to make a diagnosis even when no illness is present than to pass an ill patient as fit and well. Not only is there a pressure from colleagues to make a diagnosis, patients also are increasingly unwilling to accept less than a definite diagnosis, however senseless the label may be. The story is told of a patient who complained of a red painful tongue, and when told that he had glossitis he thanked his doctor profusely saying how much better he felt now that he knew what the problem was.

Studies in general practice have shown that the eventual outcome is the same when patients, in whom there was no definite diagnosis, were either given a symptomatic diagnosis and some medicine, or simply told that there was no evidence of any disease and therefore no need for treatment.[14] Despite the similarity in eventual outcome, a confident positive approach, even if this involved no treatment, was found to be more acceptable to patients. Some doctors find it difficult to be positive when they feel uncertain as to the cause of the illness. Others have no difficulty in attributing the illness to a viral infection, but feel the need to support this diagnosis inappropriately with antibiotics. Whatever strategem is developed to cope with this uncertainty, the patient's desire for a diagnosis influences the degree to which illness is investigated.

With the various pressures on a doctor to come up with some diagnosis, it is not surprising that the labels given to patients' illnesses are sometimes inappropriate with no scientific justification. In some cases the diseases themselves are fallacious. Shortly after radiological techniques for examining internal organs were introduced, there was a fashion for diagnosing visceroptosis of various sorts. Symptoms were attributed to stomach, kidney or colon lying too low in the abdomen. Anatomical knowledge had been derived from corpses in the supine position, and when X-rays were taken in the standing position it should have been foreseen that their position was lower than expected. However it was not, and this led to various operations to elevate the organs which, not surprisingly, had little effect on the symptoms. In some respects this concept provided one of the more notable medical successes in that the disease was eliminated when it was decided that it no longer existed!

I am indebted to Skrabanek and McCormick[15] for this description of what must be one of the more bizarre non-diseases in existence:

'The disease in question is koro, a Javanese word for the head of the turtle, a particularly intriguing, and certainly distressing, non-disease. The disease is popular in Malaysia and in South China, where it is known as suck young or shook yang, shrinking penis. According to the local experts who held a seminar during a koro epidemic in 1967, the disease is due to fear, rumour-mongering, climatic conditions and imbalance between heart and kidney. Patients afflicted by this dreadful malady live in mortal fear of dying and try to prevent the final disappearance of the penis into the abdomen by holding it with clamps, chopsticks, clothes pegs, etc., even a safety pin. In some instances the relatives take turns to hold on to the penis and sometimes the wife is asked to keep the penis in her mouth to reduce the patient's fear. Another, hardly less exotic treatment, is burning the underpants of someone of the opposite sex and using the ashes in a way unspecified.'

Too zealous an approach to the diagnostic process can lead to other potential pitfalls. It is, for example, easy to over-interpret physical findings, such as early clubbing in elderly patients with curved nails, which can then be responsible for inappropriate diagnoses. There is also a tendency to attribute symptoms to some abnormality such as a cervical rib when the evidence for the connection may be virtually non-existent. Other irrelevant findings such as a high uric acid in asymptomatic people can lead to inappropriate concern and treatment. Patients are also prone to this weakness and may develop non-side effects to a drug, particularly when problems have been reported in the media.

There is, no doubt, potential for harm in the diagnostic process. A diagnosis categorizes a person as a patient, a process which may lead to them adopting a 'sick role', but without a diagnostic label it may be difficult to be convincingly ill. Sickness can become a way of life with implications for employment and happiness; an incorrect diagnosis can then have serious repercussions. A study of steel workers, labelled as hypertensive on the basis of a diastolic pressure greater than 95 mmHg, showed increased absenteeism and decreased psychological wellbeing compared with people unaware of their hypertension.[16] In this case the findings were independent of the effect of anti-hypertensive medication, but in many cases the treatment has significant side effects, which makes it particularly important to attach the correct diagnostic label.

Most tests incur some physical risk and investigation of a patient often causes anxiety. A balance has to be struck between the cost—physical, emotional and financial—of further investigation and the benefit which might accrue from treatment of the suspected illness. There is little point in over-investigating a patient to exclude an improbable diagnosis when no treatment is available for that condition. However, the risk of not making a diagnosis of a treatable condition, however rare it might be, has also to be taken into account. In these circumstances we intuitively apply what has been called the minimax loss principle in decision theory. This minimizes the maximum loss by selecting a strategy which has the least ill effect if the worst happens. More colloquially, Feinstein[17] calls this the 'chagrin factor', a mechanism for avoiding major errors. This could lead to a test being performed to exclude an improbable diagnosis because it could seriously affect the outcome if the diagnosis was missed. Many patients with chest pain are admitted to hospital for this reason, even when the probability of myocardial infarction is low.

Despite the potential dangers and pitfalls in a diagnostic approach to medicine, there can be little doubt that the advantages far outweigh the disadvantages. Only by knowing the diagnosis can appropriate treatment be given safely; but this should not be regarded as an end in itself, it is useful only in so far as it helps in the selection of the appropriate treatment and the assessment of the prognosis. The aim of the diagnostic process is to reduce clinical uncertainty, and in many cases this can be done with minimal investigation. In other circumstances the diagnostic problem is less easily solved and a working diagnosis may have to be accepted. Whilst the level of uncertainty is unlikely to be consciously quantified, accepting a working diagnosis entails accepting doubt. More extensive investigations may reduce the uncertainty, but the question arises as to whether the extra cost justifies the change in probability.[18] Experienced doctors are more likely to bear this burden of doubt and admit to not knowing the answer to their patient's problem. It should never be forgotten that a diagnosis is made primarily for the patient's benefit and not the doctor's; when no benefit can be seen in pursuing a diagnosis further the process should be abandoned. It would be a retrograde step, however, not to aim for a diagnosis in the first place. How else could one know if a diagnosis mattered unless a list of possible diagnoses had been considered?

HYPOTHETICO-DEDUCTIVE REASONING IN CLINICAL PRACTICE

We have seen that hypothetico-deductive reasoning is both an attractive and feasible way of problem solving, and there is good evidence that adults use this technique in solving all sorts of practical problems.[19] In this section we shall be looking particularly at the evidence that hypothetico-deductive reasoning is used in the diagnostic process. That is not to say that all problems are solved in this way, less rational methods such as intuition and pattern recognition are also important and these methods will also be discussed later.

Methods of Evaluation

The studies which point towards the use by physicians of hypothetico-deductive methods in clinical diagnosis can be broadly classified into two types:

1. Those using patients or actors trained to present a clinical history and, in some cases, physical findings.[20-23] In some of these studies the doctor has been interrupted at various stages of the interview and asked for his current thoughts and reasons for asking particular questions. Clearly, a major disadvantage of this method is that the diagnostic process could be significantly altered by this disruption.

   In some studies the interview with the patient was video-taped or simply observed by the research worker for discussion later. This avoids the disruption but presents a new problem, namely difficulty in recalling the exact thought processes in retrospect.
2. Those using case vignettes presented in a variety of ways, and this includes analysis of thinking involved in clinico-pathological conferences.[21,24,25] This type of study is open to the criticism that the thinking process used in these circumstances may not be the same as those used in the presence of a patient. This raises the point that the thinking process may differ according to the circumstance and type of problem.

Hypothesis Generation and the Use of Cues

Despite the limitation of these studies, and their differences in approach, the findings have been broadly similar. Doctors, and students for that matter, do generate hypotheses, and do so early on during the interview with the patient, usually in the first few minutes. Doctors working in hospital practice will recognize that several hypotheses may be generated even before the patient is seen, on the basis of information given in the referral letter. The age, sex and main complaints will often be enough to allow the physician to form a list of possible diagnoses, the most likely diagnosis being strongly influenced by the probability of a particular disease in someone of that age and sex. A young patient with persistent bloody diarrhoea is more likely to have inflammatory bowel disease than an old patient with similar symptoms, who is more likely to have a colonic neoplasm, although both diagnoses are possible in young and old.

The number of hypotheses generated in the diagnostic process varies, but is commonly between four and seven. At any one time it is unlikely that people can consider more than three to four hypotheses, and in this respect a catch-all category can be important.[26] This may be simply an 'or something else' category, but this serves as a deposit from which new hypotheses can be generated if the findings do not adequately fit one of the original differential diagnoses. Once a diagnosis seems likely there is a risk of rigidity of thinking, and at this stage exploration of the catch-all category may provide a useful check.

In the generation of hypotheses, the importance attached to information is inappropriate in several circumstances. For example, cues discovered early on in an interview are given more emphasis in coming to a diagnosis than the same cues given later in the history. There is a danger of becoming fixed on a particular diagnosis leading to a premature closure of options. There is also a danger that the information sought may be influenced by the hypothesis considered, with the potential risk of overlooking or not seeking information which may be of crucial importance. In other words there is a risk of fixing on a hypothesis too early, thus affecting the interpretation and search for new findings. This weakness in the thought process is encapsulated in the saying, 'Don't confuse me with facts, my mind is already made up.'

A further example of misuse of information demonstrated by these studies is a tendency to over-emphasize positive findings when a negative finding may contain just as much information. This suggests that we prefer evidence that proves rather than disproves a hypothesis, whatever we should do in theory. Normal findings tend to be ignored when judging the effect of a test on the likelihood of disease.[27] When a test is performed to confirm the diagnosis of a disease and is positive, the result is taken to mean that the diagnosis is likely to be correct. A negative test should have the converse effect of making the diagnosis less likely, and yet the clinician often ignores this evidence.

A few clinical features give unequivocal information falling into one of the following categories.

1. *Pathognomonic*: the presence of such a feature guarantees the diagnosis of a particular disease. In many cases this is because the disease is defined in terms of this particular feature; e.g. a diagnosis of diabetes is defined in terms of the level of blood sugar.
2. *Exclusionary*: the finding of such a feature excludes the possibility of disease; e.g. a normal blood calcium excludes the possibility of hypercalcaemia. This type of finding is obviously the negative of pathognomonic.
3. *Obligatory*: refers to a feature which has to be present for the diagnosis of the disease, but its presence does not guarantee the diagnosis. The same finding may be present in more than one disease; e.g. airway narrowing, as shown by a reduced peak flow, has to be present for a diagnosis of acute asthma, but would also be found in other respiratory diseases.

Most findings do not confirm or exclude a diagnosis with absolute certainty. A particular clinical feature may make a diagnosis more or less likely, but doctors are not good at grading the importance of such information. We tend to think in a three point scale with cues supporting the hypothesis, refuting the hypothesis, or not influencing the diagnosis at all. In this respect computer manipulation of data is potentially more powerful, as long as the weight which should be attached to information is known. Despite this weakness in assessing the importance of information, it has been shown that failure to come to a diagnosis is usually due to a failure to consider the correct diagnosis in the first place, and not that of putting inappropriate emphasis on particular clinical findings.

Pivotal Features

It is well recognized that too much information can obscure an issue, making it difficult to see the wood for the trees. In coming to a diagnosis, it is most important to concentrate on pivotal findings or, as they have sometimes been called—lead, forceful or key features.[25] The art of picking out appropriate pivotal features may be what distinguishes an expert from a novice. Concentration on these features leads to a more parsimonious and satisfying approach to medicine. When there is a pressing need to come to a diagnosis, for example when dealing with the acutely ill patient,[23] it has been shown that doctors ask fewer questions, and whilst it could be argued that the outcome may suffer because of this, there is no evidence that it does. It is good training, in case presentations, to limit the amount of information given to encourage identification of pivotal features.

The recognition of pivotal features is not, however, always straightforward. Some findings may always be potentially serious, e.g. haematuria, but the importance of other findings may depend upon the rest of the clinical setting. Headaches may be a poor discriminatory finding, but in the presence of vomiting and confusion this feature would take on greater significance. The pivotal importance of a finding is therefore not a feature of the information itself, but depends on the context in which it is found. This makes it difficult to be didactic about the significance of a particular clinical finding, and students sometimes find this confusing.

Whilst there are some advantages in encouraging thoroughness, students should be discouraged from unnecessary data grubbing. Studies have shown that it is not so much the quantity of data which clarifies the diagnosis,[20] but rather the quality. Often there is a tendency to seek extra confirmatory findings when in fact this may add little to the original information. These extra findings may only give an illusion of validity, an example of this being dubious pallor of the optic discs in the diagnosis of multiple sclerosis. If the diagnosis is already strongly suspected this may be taken as confirmatory evidence, but the finding is likely to be discarded when there are no other features to suggest the disease. Many laboratory tests in common usage have low sensitivity and specificity, and, when the border between alternative diagnoses is unclear, additional information of this nature may only make the border fuzzier. Attempts to refine chaotic data can only lead to further chaos. Pivotal findings function like beacon lights to guide one through this fog of information.

Aggregation of Data

One way of dealing with a mass of data is to aggregate the findings whenever this is possible. Dark urine, pale stools and an itchy skin all point to a diagnosis of obstructive jaundice, and when all are present they can be considered together. A diagnosis may be made after the collection of a few clinical findings, but in the more complex cases the diagnosis can be represented by the tip of a pyramid. The main findings form the base and these may be aggregated into fewer and fewer labels as the tip is approached until the diagnosis is made. Each aggregation is like a stepping stone in the diagnostic path.

Expert vs. Novice

It is generally accepted, although not rigorously tested, that experts are better at making a diagnosis than novices, so something may be learned about the diagnostic process from studies comparing the thinking process in these two groups. One important finding is that students think in the same sort of way as experts, i.e. by generating hypotheses and testing them,[28] despite being mistakenly discouraged from formulating possible diagnoses until all the data has been collected. This should not be surprising to those who believe that the hypothetico-deductive method is a natural way of solving problems. Differences do emerge, however, when the diagnostic process is looked at in detail; experts generate hypotheses earlier in their encounters with patients,[23] and these hypotheses are more likely to be correct.[24]

The greater store of knowledge which the expert has at his or her disposal is important in reaching the correct diagnosis more quickly and reliably. But, the way this knowledge is structured in the memory is as important as the depth of knowledge.[28] This depends on experience, the inter-connection between bits of knowledge being continually updated as experience accumulates. This updating can have unfortunate consequences when, for instance, a recently diagnosed rare condition leads to an unreasonably high suspicion of this condition in subsequent patients, at least until the memory of the original case fades.[31] With greater experience this type of influence is likely to diminish.

A doctor's perception of the influence of a clinical feature on the likelihood of the diagnosis is one of the major factors governing the accuracy of a diagnosis, and this depends very much on experience.[24] Even more important is the doctor's perception of the likelihood of a particular diagnosis in his own practice, the so-called prior probability. The crucial importance of this likelihood, will be explored in greater detail when Bayes' theorem is discussed (in Chapter 4) but its importance cannot be over-emphasized. Common things are common is an old Oslerean aphorism which we would all do well to remember at all times. A major advantage that an experienced doctor has is a good feel for the likelihood of a diagnosis in the particular set of patients he is dealing with. The effect of experience on perception of base rates was demonstrated in a study of diagnostic reasoning in gastroenterology.[30] Physicians were shown to be relatively consistent in their assessment of the likelihood of various diseases, and so were surgeons. However, there were significant differences between the groups, reflecting their different experiences. Despite the importance of the prior likelihood of disease on making a diagnosis, even expert clinicians fail to take full advantage of this information.[31]

Students receive a major part of their training in teaching hospitals which have a bias towards the rarer cases seen in specialized units. When they come to practise as doctors in general practice, or district general hospitals, the likelihood of seeing these cases drops significantly. Their tendency to think of a rare disease, rather than a common one, is therefore a handicap but it will correct with time as knowledge is restructured in the memory. Some, perhaps overawed by the authority of their teachers, are reluctant to allow this restructuring to take place and thereby adapt slowly.

The ability to attach correct weights to cues is another important aspect of experience. The importance of a particular clinical finding is rarely defined in textbooks. It may be stated that the finding occurs commonly, sometimes, rarely, or even 'not uncommonly', an unnecessarily tortuous phrase, but seldom is the incidence quoted more accurately than that. In many cases there are good reasons for this. Sometimes the incidence is simply unknown, or published figures may vary widely. Arguably a more important reason is that the relevance of a clinical finding depends on the presence or absence of other clinical features. Clinical features are rarely mutually independent, the importance of one finding depending upon the presence or absence of others, as previously mentioned. It is inappropriate to state the probability of a diagnosis given the presence of a clinical feature without taking into account the other findings. This is a major problem in the application of Bayes' theorem to clinical practice, because the assumption is made that the clinical findings are independent. It also makes nonsense of examination questions such as, 'Does symptom A occur in 45%, 55% or 65% of patients with disease B?' The experienced doctor will not be able to quote the exact probability of disease when a clinical finding is present, but his experience allows of a more informed guess.

The Gathering of Clinical Information

It is still common practice for medical students to be taught to collect all the clinical information from a history and examination of the patient before formulating a list of diagnostic possibilities. This goes against the natural hypothetico-deductive method of reasoning; whilst this thoroughness has something to commend it, the blind collection of data should be discouraged. There are certainly times when a full record is useful, for example, when the legal profession is involved in a case, for if there is one word which does not enter the vocabulary of this profession, it is parsimony. A full record may also be useful to pick up incidental diseases which need attention, and, for the student, familiarity with a range of normal findings will prove useful in assessing abnormal features. But, it should be stressed that lack of thoroughness in gathering data is not as important a source of error in diagnosis as weakness in interpreting and judging information.[21]

The major disadvantage of this blunderbuss approach is the time it takes to collect all the data, much of which will not help in the diagnosis and management of the patient. A hypothesis orientated approach is both more efficient and stimulating, with emphasis being put on those features of particular relevance to the case. This economy of effort should not, however, be taken to an extreme. Time spent putting a patient at ease is not wasted;

in one study one-third of a doctor's time was spent on routine questions aimed at generating rapport and also giving time for the physician to think.[20] The latter should not be under-estimated. I remember being puzzled when one of my senior colleagues spent what seemed to be an inordinate length of time listening to someone's chest. On asking him what he could hear that I had evidently missed, he pointed out there was nothing wrong with the chest, but he needed a bit of time to think! Such honesty is not always forthcoming.

In the majority of cases, what the patient has to say about his illness—the history—contributes most to the diagnosis. In a medical out-patients setting it was shown that the final diagnosis was made on the basis of the history in 66 out of 80 patients.[32] The clinical examination and laboratory results contributed approximately equally to the diagnosis in the other cases. Clearly, the situation is likely to be different in a surgical clinic or a casualty department, but the history still remains of paramount importance in most cases.

On starting the diagnostic trail the first thing to establish is the main symptom which is concerning the patient. This is very likely to be one of the pivotal findings. Occasionally the patient does not come straight to the point, and may even obscure the issue out of embarrassment or fear, but the experienced doctor should be able to discover the main complaint quickly. Details of this presenting symptom should then be explored. For example, chest pain may be the presenting feature, but the nature of this pain must be clarified for the diagnosis to become established. This process should be one of generating hypotheses, and then trying to eliminate or confirm each one by further questioning. If the pain is described as a tight band around the chest coming on with exertion and radiating to the left arm, the diagnosis is likely to be angina. On the other hand, if the pain is limited to one side of the chest, and is worse on breathing in, the cause is more likely to be pleurisy. Once the symptoms have been aggregated under a label such as pleurisy, further questions are directed at distinguishing between the causes. If the patient had had a recent operation, and is particularly short of breath with haemoptysis, the diagnosis will almost certainly be pulmonary embolism. In the absence of these clinical features and cough, the pain may not be true pleurisy, and could be muscular. The history does not necessarily give the diagnosis, but should reduce the possibilities considerably. The aim of examination and, if needed, investigation is to clarify the situation further.

In some cases the diagnosis is not at all obvious and there may even be difficulty in thinking of an illness which could explain the clinical features. Techniques which may help in these circumstances include:

1. Listing the possible causes of the pivotal findings. This discipline is sometimes useful in thinking of diseases which could otherwise be overlooked. A junior doctor who is studying for examinations is more likely to find this useful than a senior doctor whose memory of lists will have faded.
2. Considering the possible organs in which disease could cause the main complaint. This requires only an elementary knowledge of anatomy. If the patient has a pain in the right upper quadrant of the abdomen it could be due to disease in the gall bladder, liver, kidney or colon. If this seems unlikely, other anatomical structures may also need to be considered, such as the nearby pleura, peritoneum or pancreas.
3. Thinking of the pathophysiological mechanisms by which a particular symptom could arise. A sudden blackout could be due to a fall in cerebral perfusion for which there are several possible causes, e.g. a faint, dysrhythmia, or obstruction of the vertebro-basilar circulation. Alternatively, it could be due to a sudden overwhelming electrical discharge in the brain, i.e. a fit. Hypoglycaemia may also be considered, but is much less likely when the loss of consciousness is sudden.
4. Scanning a list of disease processes in the hope of unearthing something which could explain the symptoms. This will include considering congenital, metabolic, neoplastic, infective, iatrogenic, degenerative, vasculitic, nutritional deficiencies and allergic causes.

Any or all of these techniques could be used in the hope of jogging the memory. As likely as not a doctor will know of the disease from which a patient is suffering, but has failed to think of it.

Discovering the pivotal features of the case is the most important part of history taking, but there are several other aspects which form part of routine practice as taught to medical students. Some of these aspects are aimed at the management of the patient rather than the diagnosis, and this is clearly important. The social and drug history fall largely into this category, although they can also be important in determining the diagnosis. The past history may be relevant to the current problem, but there is little point in wasting time trying to make the patient recall the exact date of his appendicectomy. Taking a full family history can be exhausting to both the patient and doctor, and in most cases would be irrelevant. If the pivotal features point towards the possible importance of a family history of disease, then questions about this become more relevant. A history of ataxia in a young person should prompt an enquiry into similar symptoms in relatives. However, without a lead from the pivotal features, family history is largely irrelevant. The discovery that a patient has a family history of diabetes does increase the likelihood of this condition, but is unlikely to strongly influence whether one specifically tests for it.

Perhaps one of the most controversial aspects of history taking is the review of symptoms. Some have argued eloquently that it should be abandoned,[33] and others believe that it is essential. It is still commonly taught as an essential part of the diagnostic process in standard textbooks of clinical skills. Undoubtedly it will occasionally turn up something of interest and possible importance, but it is time consuming and detracts from the main thrust of diagnostic thinking. Important aspects of the case should have been revealed by exploring possible causes of the patient's main problem using the hypothetico-deductive methods described. In any case it is not clear which are the main useful questions to ask routinely, and without some guidelines the review of symptoms can become extremely time consuming. Most doctors soon learn to stop routinely asking patients about their bowels and dizzy spells. Thoroughness may be a laudable maxim, but even the enthusiast should draw a line at masochism. Enthusiasts for retaining a review of symptoms should ask themselves how often, in their experience, this has led to recognition of a clinical feature which has materially influenced the diagnosis or management of a patient.

A similar argument applies to routine examination of systems. Not only can this waste time, it may also cause embarrassment. A stronger argument could be made out for a student or inexperienced doctor routinely examining all systems if time allows, but in this case this would be specifically for the purpose of gaining experience of the full range of normal variability. This is acceptable, providing that it does not inconvenience the patient, and as long as the doctor in training recognizes the reason for doing a full examination and does not feel that it is an essential part of the diagnostic process.

Accuracy of Clinical Findings

However accurate the diagnostic process may be, when the clinical findings are inaccurate a correct diagnosis may not be made. Students desperately listening for reverse splitting of the second heart sound may be unaware that even cardiologists disagree about the findings on auscultation, and specialists in other fields show an even greater disagreement when examining the heart. The assumption is made that the specialist is right, and he is usually in the privileged position of having the last say. When the chief cardiologist hears a quiet murmur there tends to be a mini-epidemic confirming it which spreads rapidly through the ranks of junior staff and students. This phenomenon, the emperor's clothes syndrome, is closely associated with terms such as very soft or intermittent murmur.[34]

Fletcher[35] was one of the first doctors to question the accuracy of clinical findings by putting this to the test. He arranged for eight experienced doctors to examine the chest of patients with emphysema to assess consistency in the evaluation of physical signs. Agreement was not very good, and, with many signs, little better than chance. He subsequently urged physicians to abandon unreliable methods and to stop teaching them to students. All doctors and students should concentrate on physical findings which are reliable and useful. How many experienced doctors use tactile fremitus, except to teach it to students?

Garland[36] and Koran[37,38] reviewed the reliability of clinical methods, data and judgement and found them all wanting. To make matters worse much of the agreement found is simply due to chance; this depends on the proportion of cases which have an abnormal finding. If two physicians each consider that half the cases have an abnormal finding, they will agree in 25% of cases by chance alone. The greater the proportion of cases considered to be abnormal the higher is the percentage agreed by chance. An overall agreement rate of 90%, with 45% agreed to be normal and 45% agreed to be abnormal, is more easily achieved than correct agreement of 85% normal and 5% abnormal.

Disagreement is not limited to clinical features found on physical examination; observer error in taking the medical history has also been shown. Cochrane and Garland[39] evaluated the agreement in symptoms recorded when coal miners were asked about their chest symptoms by four physicians. The response varied considerably, e.g. sputum 13–42%, cough 23–40%, dyspnoea 10–18% and pain 6–17%, the history recorded being influenced by the attitude of the doctor. Any doctor will have been struck by the ability of patients to give what seems to be a completely different history to different people, and even to the same person at different times. This is usually not cussedness on the part of the patient, but is a response to the way the questions are asked.

The interpretation of diagnostic procedures is also open to error. This must be immediately apparent to anyone attending X-ray meetings, and as one might expect, it applies also to interpretation of ECG, EEG and isotope studies as well as endoscopy findings. Some authors admitted to being shocked to discover that disagreement was so great among their expert miniature X-ray readers and some found this dispiriting. But we must continue to evaluate our practices objectively; the alternative is to ignore the truth for the sake of false security; that would be the antithesis of a scientific approach to medicine. Anyone interested in the literature on observer variability should refer to the extensive bibliography collected by Feinstein.[40]

What the various studies concerning the reliability of clinical signs have shown are, for the most part, not surprising. Agreement concerning the presence or absence of a sign is usually more consistent than judgement regarding continuous or qualitative variables. The more severe an abnormality the greater is the disagreement, and there is higher agreement about normality than abnormality. An encouraging finding is that judgement made by experts in their own specialty shows greater reliability than opinions of non-experts.

A distinction should be made between the consistency of observations, and their accuracy when compared with an accepted gold standard. However, one of the difficulties in judging the accuracy of clinical findings is defining a gold standard to which the clinical findings can be compared. Two physicians could agree about splenomegaly only to find that both were wrong when the spleen is examined at post-mortem. A venogram is often taken as the gold standard for the diagnosis of deep venous thrombosis, and when the clinical diagnosis of deep venous thrombosis is compared with a diagnosis based on a venogram the clinical diagnosis is little better than random.[41] However, a venogram can be difficult to interpret making it a tarnished standard. Histological data is often taken to be the ultimate gold standard, but the process of making a histological diagnosis is very much one of recognizing images and patterns, and may be just as prone to errors as a diagnosis made from clinical findings. When a histological opinion is subjected to the same critical appraisal which has been applied to clinical findings, similar disagreements have been shown.[40] There is also the added consideration of the costs of discomfort and risks incurred in obtaining tissue for histological diagnosis.

There is a tradition that when a patient dies, the post mortem is the final arbitrator as to the cause of death. It should certainly be easier to make a definite diagnosis at post mortem rather than from clinical examination and non-invasive tests before death, but with the recent advances in imaging techniques, details of pathological anatomy can be seen more readily in the living person than was possible a few decades ago. In my experience it is unusual for a post-mortem examination to reveal a surprising diagnosis when a case has been adequately investigated. More often the exact cause of death in a puzzling case remains a puzzle after the post mortem, although bronchopneumonia is a convenient label to put on the death certificate.

THE COGNITIVE CONTINUUM

The generation and testing of hypotheses by the method

described in this chapter is essentially a rational process with a thorough scientific and philosophical pedigree. Evidence has been presented which shows that physicians do use it in the diagnostic process but alternative cognitive processes can be used. The experienced doctor in particular does not sit down and consciously list a series of possible hypotheses for every patient. Usually the time is not available to do this, nor is it essential when the diagnosis is obvious. He uses the process of intuition or pattern recognition, both of which are ill-understood and possibly related.

Psychologists recognize a range of thinking processes from the intuitive to the rational and have called this the cognitive continuum.[42] Intermediate modes of thinking include the use of system aided judgement such as medical decision analysis which is explored later in this book. First let us look at the two main influences on the type of thinking processes used to solve medical problems:

1. Hammond and co-workers[43] considered the most important influence on the thinking process to be the nature of the problem. Intuitive thinking is favoured when there are many cues available or strong pivotal signs. A patient showing the classical features of thyrotoxicosis can be diagnosed readily without conscious listing of possible diagnoses. Even so, there can be few doctors who would not test their diagnosis by performing thyroid function tests. In contrast to this, when quantitative data is available an analytical process is more likely to be used, particularly if there is a clear analytical path to follow.

2. Hubert and Stuart Dreyfus[44] argued that experience was more important than the task in hand in determining the thinking process used. The novice cannot rely on experience to recognize patterns of disease and must think analytically to avoid errors. This also applies to the experienced doctor when dealing with unfamiliar problems, and there is some evidence that this happens. On the other hand, the experienced doctor looking at familiar problems is more likely to use intuitive methods.

Intuitive and analytical reasoning are not mutually exclusive. The generation of a hypothesis may be largely intuitive, but it can still be subjected to analytical reason when tested. The diagnosis which first comes to mind may fit the clinical pattern so well that other diagnoses need not be seriously considered. The confident recognition of varicose veins does not require much experience, so the problem of generating a list of possible diagnoses does not arise. However, when the clinical features do not adequately fit any disease, even the experienced physician will need to carefully consider all the possibilities and eliminate those diagnoses which seem less likely.

The exact nature of the intuitive process, which is clearly important in the diagnostic process as used by the experts, is poorly understood. It is possible to envisage the rapid application of a hypothetico-deductive method without a list of possible diagnoses being made at the conscious level. A radiologist may detect an abnormality on an X-ray film and, without consciously considering the possible causes, seek further clues to substantiate a possible diagnosis or build up a pattern which can be accepted as consistent with a particular disease. With experience, no detached choice or deliberation occurs. An expert driver is not conscious of driving his car, and yet can respond to an emergency more appropriately than a learner. Indeed, he may respond better for not analysing the situation. When faced with a vehicle pulling out in front of him, he does not consciously compute the relative risks of applying the breaks or swerving to avoid it. From previous experience an unconscious prediction as to the relative risk of these choices is made and the appropriate action taken. To try and consciously rationalize the situation could well literally prove fatal.

Similarly for the diagnostic process, it is the doctor experienced in the task in hand who is more likely to use intuitive methods with a resulting advantage of speed. Analytical methods are slower but potentially more accurate particularly for the more complicated cases. Nevertheless, it is as well to remember that whilst experience can be the mainstay of diagnostic skill, over-reliance on it can lead to nothing more than making the same mistake with increasing confidence.

Exactly how pattern recognition relates to the intuitive process is unclear, but it is a non-rational process more safely used by the doctor who has considerable experience of disease presenting in different ways. A certain set of clinical features may obviously point to a diagnosis as soon as a patient enters the consulting room, e.g. Parkinsonism and hypothyroidism, but there are not many instances where the main clinical features are apparent immediately. In most cases the clinical features have to be sought and the seeking of these features should, and usually does, involve the generation of hypotheses along with the deduction of consequences and testing of these from the history, examination and investigations.

Medical students are taught a systematic analytical approach to diagnosis, and this is entirely appropriate in view of their inexperience. They may, however, feel that their teachers are applying double standards when they see them using intuitive methods in their routine clinical practice. It should now be clear that this is not as inconsistent as it may at first appear to be, and if medical students are aware of the full range of cognitive processes used in making a diagnosis it should help them to change their thinking processes as experience allows.

FURTHER READING

Balla, J. I. *The Diagnostic Process*. Cambridge: Cambridge University Press, 1985.

Dowie, J. and Elstein, A. (eds). *Professional Judgement*. Cambridge: Cambridge University Press, 1988.

Elstein, A., Shulman, L. S. and Sprafka, S. A. *Medical Problem Solving: an Analysis of Clinical Reasoning*. Cambridge, Mass.: Harvard University Press, 1978.

Gale, J. and Marsden, P. *Medical Diagnosis*. Oxford: Oxford University Press, 1983.

Kassirer, J. P. Diagnostic reasoning. *Annals of Internal Medicine* 1989; **110**: 897–900.

Riegelman, R. K. *Minimizing Medical Mistakes: The Art of Medical Decision Making*. Boston: Little Brown and Co., 1991.

4

Evaluation of Tests

'Before ordering a test decide what you will do if it is (a) positive or (b) negative, and if both answers are the same don't do the test.'

Archie Cochrane

INTRODUCTION

It is often possible to make a diagnosis from the clinical history and physical examination, but unacceptable doubt about the diagnosis may remain unless ancillary tests are undertaken. There are now many such tests available, most of these having been developed in this century, and they range from simple urine tests to complicated computer imaging. It is easy to be bedazzled by the sophistication of the technology, but the interpretation of tests can be beset with pitfalls for the unwary. An ideal test is one that gives an unequivocal answer which confirms or disproves a possible diagnosis, but this rarely happens except when the disease is defined in terms of the test, and even then the doctor is at the mercy of laboratory errors. The great majority of tests, whatever their nature, do not give a precise answer, although some, as might be expected, are better than others. In this chapter the basic rules which govern the limits of certainty will be applied to the use of laboratory tests and other investigations.

The problem is that of defining the probability of a diagnosis when a test result is either positive or negative. In statistical terms this is called a conditional probability and involves two events; the occurrence of the second, in this case the diagnosis, depending on the occurrence of the first, the test result. The rules governing this were discovered by Thomas Bayes, an 18th century English Presbyterian minister from Tunbridge Wells; these rules would have been lost were it not for their discovery by his relatives on sorting out his papers after his death. Ledley and Lusted (1959)[45] appear to have been the first people to apply the rules to medical problems.

Anyone interested in the derivation of Bayes' formula can find this in the appendix at the end of this chapter. It is not essential to know this to follow the use of the theorem, but since it requires only an elementary knowledge of algebra to understand, the effort to do so may be worthwhile if only to eliminate the mystique surrounding it. In any case a knowledge of the simple notation used is necessary to understand both the derivation and the application of Bayes' theorem so the following should be read first.

BAYES' THEOREM: NOTATION

We are interested in knowing the probability of a diagnosis when a test is positive. This statement in Bayesian notation is written as follows:

$$P(D|F)$$

D stands for diagnosis and F for finding; the line between them is read as 'given that'. Therefore, the above formula is read as, 'The probability of a diagnosis given the finding'. This is precisely what we require in clinical practice.

In its simplest form Bayes' formula states that:

$$P(D|F) = \frac{P(D) \cdot P(F|D)}{P(F)} \qquad (1)$$

The probability of the diagnosis in question, $P(D)$, refers to the likelihood of the diagnosis in the particular population to which the test is being applied. This is one of the important practical limitations of the theorem; $P(D)$ differs according to the type of patient the doctor normally deals with. The likelihood of finding a patient with Cushing's disease is very different in general practice compared with an endocrinology clinic.

P(F|D) is the probability of a specific finding when a group of patients with that diagnosis are studied, e.g. the proportion of patients with acute leukaemia who have splenomegaly. This type of data should be available from the literature.

P(F) is the likelihood of the finding being present in the type of patient seen. Again this will depend on the practice of the doctor—patients with splenomegaly are relatively commonly seen in haematological practice. Some of these patients will have leukaemia and some will not. The overall probability of finding an enlarged spleen is thus comprised of the chance of finding splenomegaly in patients with leukaemia and the chance of finding splenomegaly in patients who do not have leukaemia; in the context of making a diagnosis of leukaemia these are regarded as false positives.

In Bayesian notation this is written as:

$$P(F) = P(D) \cdot P(F|D) + P(\overline{D}) \cdot P(F|\overline{D}) \qquad (2)$$

The notation for the absence of a disease is $\overline{D}$. The term $P(D) \cdot P(F|D)$ refers to the patients who have splenomegaly and leukaemia, whereas $P(\overline{D}) \cdot P(F|\overline{D})$ refers to the patients who do not have leukaemia but who, nevertheless, have splenomegaly.

Bayes' theorem is often used in the slightly more forbidding form:

$$P(D|F) = \frac{P(D) \cdot P(F|D)}{P(D) \cdot P(F|D) + P(\overline{D}) \cdot P(F|\overline{D})} \qquad (3)$$

This is often easier to use in practice than equation (1), and simply follows from combining equations (1) and (2). Equation (1) is useful, though, for emphasizing the two fundamental implications of the theorem:

1. P(D), which is called the prior probability of the diagnosis in the population studied, i.e. the probability before the test is applied, is crucial in determining the probability of the disease when the test is positive, P (D|F). A failure to appreciate the importance of prior probability can lead to an inexperienced doctor putting undue emphasis on a positive investigation.

2. The P(F|D) is changed to P(D|F). Data is often expressed in the form P(F|D); e.g. in the standard textbook the disease is specified in the title of the chapter, and the findings, given the disease, then described. In practice, the patient presents not with the disease, but with a set of clinical features and the challenge is to determine the chance of a particular disease given those findings, i.e. P(D|F). This theorem allows this transition to be made.

APPLICATION OF BAYES' THEOREM

The potential for using Bayes' theorem in medical practice is considerable, but the principles are particularly useful when applied to the influence of a single test result on the likelihood of a patient having a certain disease. In this section two simple examples will be taken to show the usefulness and power of the theorem applied in this way. However, care should be taken not to use the theorem too enthusiastically because of problems and pitfalls which exist. An outline of these will be considered in the final section of this chapter.

The first example concerns the usefulness of a positive antineutrophil cytoplasmic antibody test (ANCA) in the diagnosis of Wegener's granulomatosis. The ANCA test seems to be relatively accurate in the diagnosis of Wegener's granulomatosis. In 100 patients with this condition you can expect the test to be positive in approximately 80, but false positive results also occur. In 100 patients who do not have this disease about 2 will have a positive test, i.e.

$$P(F|D) = 0.80$$

$$P(F|\overline{D}) = 0.02$$

If this test is applied to a group of patients in whom you assess their chance of having Wegener's granulomatosis to be 30%, i.e.

$$P(D) = 0.30$$

the significance of a positive finding would be as follows:

$$P(D|F) = \frac{P(D) \cdot P(F|D)}{P(D) \cdot P(F|D) + P(\overline{D}) \cdot P(F|\overline{D})}$$

$$P(D|F) = \frac{(0.3)(0.8)}{(0.3)(0.8) + (0.7)(0.02)}$$

$$P(D|F) = 0.95$$

The consequences of a positive test are:

1. The probability of Wegener's granulomatosis has been changed from a prior probability of 0.30 to a probability of 0.95. This is a very significant change in the likelihood of disease but, inevitably with any imperfect test, some doubt remains.
2. The probability of a diagnosis given a finding, $P(D|F)$, has been derived from the probability of a finding given a diagnosis, $P(F|D)$.

The second example explores the usefulness of an exercise cardiograph in the diagnosis of ischaemic heart disease and takes the analysis one step further by looking at the effect of both a positive and negative result, as well as at the influence of different levels of prior probability on the final diagnosis. To do this it is first necessary to know what the probability of the diagnosis is when the test is negative, $P(D|\overline{F})$. This is given by:

$$P(D|\overline{F}) = \frac{P(D) \cdot P(\overline{F}|D)}{P(D) \cdot P(\overline{F}|D) + P(\overline{D}) \cdot P(\overline{F}|\overline{D})} \qquad (4)$$

Published work shows that out of 100 people with ischaemic heart disease as shown on angiography, approximately 64 have a positive exercise ECG, and out of 100 people with no ischaemic heart disease, 11 would have a positive exercise test[46]; i.e.

$$P(F|D) = 0.64 \qquad\qquad P(\overline{F}|D) = 0.36$$

$$P(F|\overline{D}) = 0.11 \qquad\qquad P(\overline{F}|\overline{D}) = 0.89$$

Figure 4.1 shows the results of fitting these values into Bayes' formula ((3) and (4)) at three different levels of prior probability,

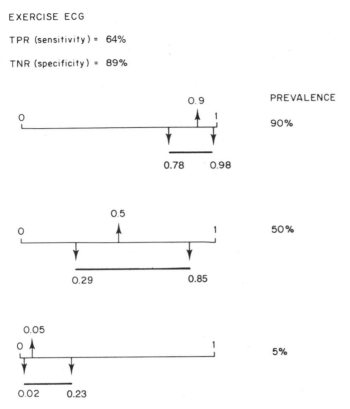

Figure 4.1 *Bayes' theorem and exercise ECG: influence of an exercise test result on the likelihood of ischaemic heart disease for three different levels of prior probability (prevalence).*

0.05, 0.5, and 0.9, which approximately fit the clinical labels of non-anginal chest pain, atypical angina and typical angina. The bar represents the discriminatory power of the test at each level of prior probability, a positive test leading to a post-test probability to the extreme right of the bar, and a negative test to a post test probability to the extreme left of the bar.

The analysis shows that the test is most useful for deciding the likelihood of ischaemic heart disease in a patient with atypical chest pain. If the diagnosis is already likely, the test may only confuse the issue by giving a false negative result; the diagnosis is still likely to be angina. Similarly, when the diagnosis is not at all likely before the test, it remains unlikely even after a positive test. An analysis of this sort highlights the type of patient for whom the test is likely to be useful, and demonstrates the potential power of Bayes' theorem when applied to medical problems. Uncertainty is not eliminated, but it can be reduced.

SPECIFICITY AND SENSITIVITY OF TESTS

Jacob Yerushalmy (1947)[47] introduced the terms sensitivity and specificity of a diagnostic test, and applied these terms to an epidemiological problem where the diagnosis was known and the accuracy of the test evaluated in retrospect. These concepts are best considered in relation to Bayes' theorem, and the terms can be directly incorporated into the formula. Although the concepts are not difficult to grasp, they can be difficult to remember. Those readers with similar difficulties to my own in this respect may take comfort from knowing that they are in good company, as I was much relieved to see a professor of statistics, on teaching this topic, take a note out of his pocket and unashamedly admit that he could never remember which was which!

The *sensitivity* of the test is the percentage of patients with a positive result from a population with the disease. This is the true positive rate (TPR) of the test or, in Bayesian notation, $P(F|D)$. A test with a high sensitivity would pick out most patients who have the disease in question.

The *specificity* of a test is the percentage of patients with a negative test in a population without disease. This is the true negative rate (TNR) of the test or $P(\overline{F}|\overline{D})$. In other words, if the specificity of a test is high a negative result virtually excludes the possibility of the diagnosis.

Some readers may find it helpful to remember that *se*nsitivity is to do with the *p*ositive rate of the test and *s*pecificity with the *n*egative rate, but others may find this even more confusing. To summarize:

$$Sensitivity = TPR = P(F|D)$$

$$Specificity = TNR = P(\overline{F}|\overline{D})$$

When a new test is first evaluated it is often used in a group of patients who are known to have the disease, and in a group of patients who are known not to have the disease. In other words, the diagnosis is already established, and because these types of sensitivity and specificity measurement are defined in terms of the disease they have been called nosological.[48]

The nature of the diseased and non-diseased groups chosen to evaluate the test can be crucial to the sensitivity and specificity derived. For example, consider the usefulness of the anti-nuclear factor, ANF, in the diagnosis of systemic lupus erythematosus (SLE). Virtually all patients with SLE would have a positive result, and very few people without significant illness would have a positive test. The test would seem to have a very high sensitivity and specificity. However, patients with SLE are not likely to be confused with people in good health. They are more likely to be confused with patients who suffer from other vasculitic disorders and these patients may well have a positive ANF. The usefulness of the test would be better assessed by comparing a group with SLE to a group with other vasculitic disorders. The specificity of the test would fall dramatically and a more specific test, e.g. antibody to double stranded DNA, will fare much better. Quoted values of sensitivity and specificity may, therefore, be of limited relevance to clinical practice unless derived from studies using appropriate groups. The relevance will also be limited to the type of patient seen in the diseased population. If the test is evaluated only in patients with extensive disease, the sensitivity measured may not apply to patients with more limited disease.

This type of sensitivity and specificity cannot be used directly to predict the likelihood of a particular patient having the disease. When faced with a patient, we are not interested in the probability of a finding given a diagnosis, $P(F|D)$, the sensitivity, but need to know the probability of a diagnosis given a finding, $P(D|F)$. The calculation of this requires knowledge of the prior probability of the disease in the particular patient tested, which can then be inserted into Bayes' formula along with the sensitivity and specificity of the test.

However, there is an alternative way of evaluating a new test which gives a different type of sensitivity and specificity directly applicable to diagnosis. This involves using a group of patients suspected of having a particular disease which the test is designed to diagnose. After full evaluation, which may include the passage of time, patients in this group are designated as having or not having the disease. It is now possible to directly interpret the relevance of a finding in that particular clinical setting by using what has sometimes been called the diagnostic sensitivity and specificity. To avoid confusion most people refer to these as the predictive value of the test.

$$\text{Diagnostic sensitivity} = \text{negative predictive value} = P(\overline{D}|\overline{F})$$

$$\text{Diagnostic specificity} = \text{positive predictive value} = P(D|F)$$

For a realistic evaluation of the test in these and other circumstances it is essential that the result of the test does not influence the diagnosis either by altering the way the diagnosis is made (work-up bias), or as a result of reviewing the interpretation of the main test which has been used to establish the diagnosis (diagnostic review bias). Similarly, the converse should not be allowed to happen, i.e. the knowledge of the diagnosis should not influence the interpretation of the test which is being evaluated (test review bias).

An example may help to illustrate the relationship between these measurements. Imagine a large series of patients with a fairly high probability of hepatocellular carcinoma, say 5%, e.g. patients with relapse of liver problems after having had hepatitis B when younger. The alphafoetoprotein test is a test for hepatocellular carcinoma which we wish to evaluate. There are 1000 patients in all and 50 patients are found, by an independent method, to have hepatocellular carcinoma. Figure 4.2 shows the number of patients with and without hepatocellular carcinoma who have a positive or negative test and the resulting sensitivity, specificity and predictive values.

The relationship between these measures of a test's usefulness is given by Bayes' theorem. A glance at equation (3) will show that the sensitivity—$P(F|D)$—and positive predictive value—$P(D|F)$—can be fitted directly into the formula, but specificity cannot. However, the false positive rate (FPR), $P(F|\overline{D})$, which appears in the formula, is related to the true negative rate, specificity, in the following way

$$\text{FPR} = 1 - \text{TNR} = 1 - \text{specificity}$$

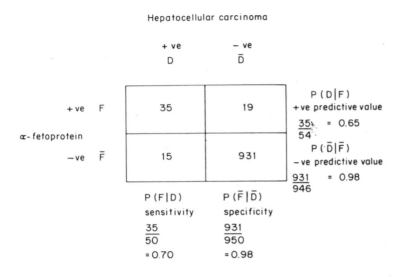

Figure 4.2 *Evaluation of the usefulness of an alphafoetoprotein test in the diagnosis of hepatocellular carcinoma.*

so Bayes' formula becomes:

$$\frac{\text{positive predictive}}{\text{value}} = \frac{P(D) \cdot \text{sensitivity}}{P(D) \cdot \text{sensitivity} + P(\overline{D}) \cdot (1 - \text{specificity})}$$

This again emphasizes that the real predictive value of a test, and, therefore, its usefulness, depends upon the likelihood of the diagnosis, P(D), in the population to which it is applied. If the alphafoetoprotein test was used to check for hepatocellular carcinoma in all patients with any form of liver disease, the number of false positives would be so high that the test would be valueless. The reader may like to calculate the positive predictive value of the test in different populations. If, for example, the probability of hepatocellular carcinoma was only P=0.01, the positive predictive value would be 0.26. For every true positive result there would be three false positive ones. A screening test used in a predominantly normal population would have to have a very high sensitivity and specificity to pick out the majority of people with the disease in question while avoiding undue waste of resources and unnecessary anxiety from false positive results. In this respect mammography is not a particularly good screening test because the positive predictive value in asymptomatic people is relatively low. The emotional stress, physical risk and financial costs that this entails has not stopped its widespread use.

This point is so important that it is worth emphasizing. Forget about formulae for a minute and just look at some simple figures. Imagine a test for lung cancer which gives a false positive rate of 10% (specificity=0.9). If this is applied to an adult population with a prevalence of lung cancer of 100 in 100 000, then

100 have lung cancer

99 900 do not have lung cancer

Of the patients who do not have lung cancer, 10%, i.e. 9990, would have a false positive result. The implications of this are enormous.

EFFICIENCY OF DIAGNOSTIC TESTS

It follows from what has been said that the efficiency of a diagnostic test depends upon

1. Sensitivity of the test.
2. Specificity of the test.
3. The prevalence of the disease in the population to which the test is applied.

The relationship between these three variables is given by

$$\text{Efficiency} = \frac{\text{TP results} + \text{TN results}}{\text{total no. results}}$$

$$= \frac{N \cdot P(D) \cdot \text{sensitivity} + N \cdot P(\overline{D}) \cdot \text{specificity}}{N}$$

$$= P(D) \cdot \text{sensitivity} + P(\overline{D}) \cdot \text{specificity}$$

If prevalence, $P(D)$, is high, the efficiency of a test is most influenced by the sensitivity, and when the prevalence is low, the specificity is particularly important.

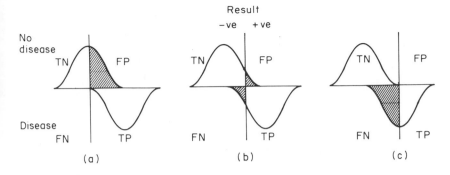

Figure 4.3 *Influence of choosing different cut-off points between positive and negative results. Normal distributions of a continuous variable for people with and without the disease are shown.*

When the result of a test is graded as, for example, it is with most biochemical tests, the sensitivity and specificity of the test can be altered by moving the cut-off point which is regarded as the division between normality and abnormality (Figure 4.3). The number of false positive results (FP) will vary according to where the line is drawn, and this can be altered to suit the clinical problem to which the test is going to be applied. If the test is going to be used for screening a large population with a low incidence of disease, the line needs to be over to the right (Figure 4.3C) to avoid a significant proportion of false positive results. However, in doing this the negative predictive value of the test will be reduced, leading to a high number of false negative results.

Likelihood Ratios

The power of a test to discriminate between normal and abnormal can be expressed as a *likelihood ratio* (LR) and this may help in deciding where to draw the cut-off point in the circumstances depicted in Figure 4.3. The likelihood ratio is defined as follows

$$LR+ = \frac{TPR}{FPR} = \frac{P(F|D)}{P(F|\bar{D})} \text{for positive results}$$

$$LR- = \frac{FNR}{TNR} = \frac{P(\bar{F}|D)}{P(\bar{F}|\bar{D})} \text{for negative results}$$

The more the cut-off point is moved to the right in Figure 4.3 the higher the ratio of TPR/FPR becomes and, therefore, the higher is LR+. A LR+ of 10 means the diagnosis is 10 times as likely as not when the result is positive, and an LR+ equal to infinity is diagnostic. But as the cut-off point is moved to the right the ratio of FNR/TNR increases and a negative test is less useful. When the line is moved to the left the ratio of FNR/TNR approaches and eventually equals zero (Figure 4.3A) when LR− =0. A negative result would then exclude the possibility of the diagnosis. The line should be drawn in a position which best suits what is required from the test.

The reader will have appreciated how easy it is to get confused about these various terms and their relationships so for ease of reference they are summarized in Figure 4.4.

Odds

Some people prefer to think in terms of odds rather than probability and one advantage of the LRs is that they can be applied directly to change the odds ratio:

$$odds = \frac{\text{probability of event occurring}}{\text{probability of event not occurring}}$$

$$= \frac{P}{1-P}$$

$P(F\|D)$	TPR	Sensitivity
$P(\bar{F}\|\bar{D})$	TNR	Specificity
$P(\bar{F}\|D)$	FNR	
$P(F\|\bar{D})$	FPR	
$P(D\|F)$	Positive predictive value	
$P(\bar{D}\|\bar{F})$	Negative predictive value	
LR +	$\dfrac{\text{TPR}}{\text{FPR}}$	$\dfrac{\text{Sensitivity}}{1-\text{specificity}}$
LR −	$\dfrac{\text{FNR}}{\text{TNR}}$	$\dfrac{1-\text{sensitivity}}{\text{specificity}}$
Efficiency	$P(D) \cdot \text{sensitivity} + P(\bar{D}) \cdot \text{specificity}$	

Figure 4.4 *Summary of terminology used in this chapter.*

Thus, when P=0.67 the odds are 0.67/0.33 which equals 2:1. Now, the post-test odds equals pre-test odds times LR for either a positive (LR+) or negative (LR−) result. If the LR+ for a test was 6, and with these pre-test odds, the post-test odds would be 12:1 assuming, of course, that the test was positive.

Receiver Operating Characteristic Curves

Receiver operating characteristic curves,[49] or their mirror image, the performance characteristic curves,[50] can be a useful and sophisticated alternative way of deciding which cut-off point to use. Figure 4.5 shows an example of a performance characteristic curve which directly relates the sensitivity of a test to its specificity. The curve is drawn from a series of points relating the sensitivity and specificity of a test using different cut-off points as described above. It is now possible to choose a point which minimizes the number of mistakes made and this is the point where the slope of the tangent to the curve at that point is related to the prevalence as follows:

$$slope = \frac{prevalence - 1}{prevalence}$$

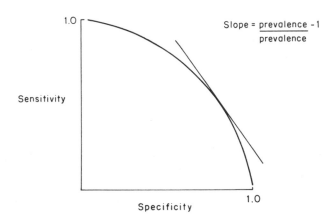

Figure 4.5 *Performance characteristic curve of a test with different cut-off points between normal and abnormal giving different sensitivities and specificities.*

This is not, however, necessarily the best point to choose. If the cost, financial or otherwise, of missing a diagnosis is high, then a test with a high sensitivity is required. The additional cost of a false positive or a false negative result, e.g. in person years or average financial cost of a person year, can be incorporated into the concept in a quantitative way. Anyone wishing to take this aspect further could start with the paper by McNeil, Keeler and Adelstein.[49]

MULTIPLE FINDINGS AND BAYES' THEOREM

So far in this chapter, Bayes' theorem has been applied to the effect of one particular finding on the probability of a specified disease, but Bayes' theorem has a much wider potential application, although there are both theoretical and practical problems accompanying its wider use. For example, consider the situation where there are several different findings, which is usual in clinical practice, and the problem is to find the probability of a particular diagnosis given a set of findings (F_s). If the clinical findings are independent of each other then

$$P(F_s|D) = P(F_1|D) \cdot P(F_2|D) \cdot P(F_3|D) \ . \ . \ . \ P(F_n|D)$$

and $P(F_s|D)$ can be inserted directly into Bayes' formula to give $P(D|F_s)$.

The problem with this simple modification is that findings are usually not independent. An obvious example of this would be the finding of pale stools and dark urine in obstructive jaundice. In other cases the connection is less obvious but still significant. The connection between anaemia and dyspnoea is fairly apparent, but the relationship between a thyroxine level and dyspnoea may be less obvious. Furthermore, when a second test is done on the basis of the result of a first test, these tests cannot be truly independent.

Bayes' theorem can deal with dependency between findings but the formula becomes complex. The term $P(F_s|D)$ takes the form

$$P(F_s|D) = P(F_1|D) \cdot P(F_2|DF_1) \cdot P(F_3|DF_1F_2) \ . \ . \ . \ P(F_n|DF_1F_2 \ . \ . \ . \ F_{n-1})$$

which makes the formula not only difficult to handle, but pre-supposes that a lot of information is available. Trying to find data on $P(F_1|D)$ is hard enough, but the reader will appreciate the difficulties in finding data such as $P(F_3|DF_1F_2)$ which is the probability of a finding—F_3—given that a patient has a diagnosis, and positive findings F_1 and F_2.

Fryback[51] discusses the problems in some depth and shows that the effect of mutual dependence of data can be quite marked, although the effect is less significant the fewer the number of variables there are. He derives a first order approximation which is simpler than the full formula, but this is still unwieldy and necessitates a lot of information which is not likely to be available. When a number of possible diseases as well as several findings are considered, Bayes' theorem can still be used, but the formula is so complex that it is not likely to be of practical benefit in the medical field.

LINEAR DISCRIMINANT FUNCTIONS

An elegant way of overcoming some of the practical problems is to use the system of weights first described by Spiegelhalter,[52] and later used in the evaluation of gastrointestinal symptoms.[53] The advantage of this approach is that each relevant clinical feature carries a certain weight of evidence. In calculating the probability of a diagnosis, all the physician has to do is to add up each weight of evidence, according to whether the feature is present or not, and then convert the sum back to a probability.

The concept is based on the use of odds and LRs in the way previously described in this chapter:

$$\text{post-test odds} = \text{pre-test odds} \cdot \text{LR}$$

Assuming independence of finding for the moment, when several findings are considered it follows that:

$$\text{post-test odds} = \text{pre-test odds} \cdot \text{LR}_1 \cdot \text{LR}_2 \ldots \cdot \text{LR}_n$$

For convenience the LRs are now converted to weights of evidence by taking the logarithm which allows them to be summated.

Taking the natural logarithm and multiplying by 100:

$$100 \log_e \text{ post odds} = 100 \log_e \text{ prior odds} + 100 \log_e LR_1 + 100 \log_e LR_2$$

$$\ldots + 100 \log_e LR_n$$

i.e. using the terminology of the method,

total score (T) = starting score + wt of evidence 1 + wt of evidence 2

$$\ldots + \text{wt of evidence n}$$

The total score can now be converted back to probability as follows:

$$\text{predicted post-test probability (\%)} = \frac{e^{T/100} \cdot 100}{1 + e^{T/100}}$$

A complication is that the laws of conditional probability only apply if the findings are mutually independent. To allow for the effect of dependence between findings, the weights of evidence have to be adjusted. This is achieved by the technique of logistic regression; whilst this makes the analysis of data from which the weights of evidence are derived more difficult, it does not complicate the use of these weights in clinical practice once they have been determined. Those readers interested in the technique should refer to the original article.[52]

The mathematics involved in this approach may seem unwieldy for routine clinical practice, but the concept of weights of evidence is both readily appreciated and attractive. Once the adjusted weights of evidence have been derived from the appropriate publications they can be used quite simply by non-mathematically inclined physicians. Each finding has a weight and the total weight is obtained by summating the weight of each finding. The conversion back to probability can be done by reference to a table. An example of the technique used for predicting post-operative respiratory complications in a group of elderly surgical patients is described in a paper by Seymour, et al.[54]

DIFFICULTIES IN APPLYING BAYES' THEOREM TO MEDICINE

Many of the difficulties the physician faces in the use of Bayes' theorem in clinical practice apply also to the implementation of decision analysis, and the speed with which the practising physician has to make decisions is one of these. Although the calculations are not particularly complex, they do take more time than is generally available. Moreover, the physician is not used to this quantitative approach to medicine, and the patient does not expect it. Not that these alone should prevent the use of the concepts, but they do need to provide clear advantages before being embraced enthusiastically. The concepts were first applied to medical problems by Ledley and Lusted in 1959 but they are still not widely used today which suggests difficulty in their implementation.

One serious problem, which is also common to decision analysis, is that the information demanded by these formal methods of analysis is often not available. Even with all the time in the world it is often impossible to find exact conditional probabilities in the literature. Textbooks may state that a finding is common or uncommon in a certain disease, but rarely is a precise figure given. Differences in the population of patients, methods of testing and expertise may mean that sensitivity and specificity from pooled data may not be applicable to the patient in your own particular practice. Accurate predictions are best made when there is a good local database, but this could take years to gather and may no longer be relevant when collected. Nevertheless, even imperfect data is infinitely preferable to no data, and one of the strengths of Bayesian statistics is that it highlights deficiency in data and points to the questions which should be asked.

Whilst the statistical validity of Bayes' theorem is well established, it should not be forgotten that the prior probability of disease is an important determinant of the final likelihood of disease. Almost invariably, in routine practice, this means making a subjective estimate which is no more than a personal guess, and often not a good one at that. When subjective estimates of prior probability were compared in a group of physicians there was very wide variance in these estimates; and when the same estimates were converted into predicted outcomes, and compared with the known outcomes, the correlation was alarmingly poor.[55] Moreover, in this study, the estimates were no better in the more experienced physicians. This points towards an urgent need for data on which objective estimates of prior probability can be made: it is ironic that by using subjective estimates, the quest for reducing uncertainty through Bayesian statistics ultimately depends on making a guess.

Nor should one forget the limits imposed by conditional independence. When a test is applied in practice, several clinical facts may already be known about the patient, and these may include the results of preliminary investigations. This determines the prior probability of disease, and the sensitivity and the specificity of a further test may be influenced by this. In other words, if sensitivity and specificity values are to be used, they should only be applied to a population similar to the one used in the evaluation of the test in the first place. The accuracy of an ultrasound examination of the liver may well be different when applied to a group of patients with weight loss, enlarged liver and a history of cancer compared to a group of patients suffering from indigestion. Moreover, when Bayes' theorem is applied to tests used sequentially, the order in which they are applied affects the sensitivity and specificity of these tests. This would apply, for example, to the accuracy of thallium scans and exercise ECG in the evaluation of ischaemic heart disease.

Despite these limitations there is a lot to be learned from the application of Bayesian statistics to medical problems. Even when a dearth of information excludes the formal use of these statistical methods the principles upon which they rely are still valid. The usefulness of an investigation will depend upon the population tested, and this should always be borne in mind. The importance of prior probability cannot be overemphasized; this, along with the sensitivity and specificity of a test, defines the limits of the test's usefulness. When a new test is developed it should be subjected to the same rigorous standards that apply to the introduction of a new drug so that the accuracy can be defined. To do otherwise can be both expensive and dangerous.

It is impossible to predict with certainty the likelihood of a diagnosis when a test is positive or negative without knowledge of the prior probability. However, it is possible to report the result of a test in such a way that the true meaning of the result can be seen in the clinical context by quoting the likelihood of a diagnosis for different prior probability levels. This should be done more frequently to encourage the physician to quantify the strength of his diagnostic suspicion.

APPENDIX: PROOF OF BAYES' THEOREM

The formal definition of conditional probability is

$$P(D|F) = \frac{P(F \& D)}{P(F)} \tag{A1}$$

This self-evident truth can be more easily appreciated in the form

$$P(F \& D) = P(F) \cdot P(D|F)$$

The probability of the finding and the disease occurring together—$P(F \& D)$—clearly depends first on the probability of the finding, and then on the probability of having the disease when the finding is positive. If 20% of the population have a positive finding and 75% of these have the disease then 15 out of 100 (75% of 20) will have both the finding and the disease.

The probability of a positive finding is the sum of the probability of the finding when the disease is present, and the probability of the positive finding when the disease is not present, i.e.

$$P(F) = P(F \& D) + P(F \& \overline{D}) \tag{A2}$$

When equation (A2) is inserted into equation (A1) the following is obtained

$$P(D|F) = \frac{P(F \& D)}{P(F \& D) + P(F \& \overline{D})} \tag{A3}$$

using the rules of conditional probability again

$$P(F|D) = \frac{P(F \& D)}{P(D)}$$

$$P(F|\overline{D}) = \frac{P(F \& \overline{D})}{P(\overline{D})}$$

These can then be substituted in equation (A3) to give

$$P(D|F) = \frac{P(D) \cdot P(F|D)}{P(D) \cdot P(F|D) + P(\overline{D}) \cdot P(F|\overline{D})} \tag{A4}$$

if the denominator of this equation is left in the original form, i.e. P(F), the equation can be seen in its simplest form.

$$P(D|F) = \frac{P(D) \cdot P(F|D)}{P(F)}$$

FURTHER READING

Feinstein, A. R. The haze of Bayes, the aerial palaces of decision analysis and the computerized ouija board. *Clinical Pharmacology and Therapeutics* 1977; **21**: 482–496.

Hopkins, A. (ed.) *Appropriate Investigation and Treatment in Clinical Practice*. London: Royal College of Physicians, 1989.

Moore, P. G. and Thomas, H. *The Anatomy of Decisions*. London: Penguin Books, 1988.

Phillips, G. (ed.) *Logic in Medicine*. London: BMJ publications, 1988.

Wulff, H. R. *Rational Diagnosis and Treatment*. Oxford: Blackwell Scientific Publications, 1981.

5
Computer Aided Diagnosis

'The heart has its reasons that reason does not know.'

Pascal

INTRODUCTION

Many aspects of health care have benefited from the introduction of computers, such as medical administration, computer assisted learning, collection of clinical data for audit, and automation of medical equipment. Computer programs have also been developed to help in the process of clinical diagnosis, and since they have the potential for solving difficult problems, they also have the potential for reducing diagnostic uncertainty. It is this aspect of computer usage which is covered in this chapter.

In the 1960s and 1970s it was hoped that computers could be developed into problem solving machines which would equal or better the ability of humans. The application of these ideas to the diagnosis and management of medical problems was an idea that was both exciting and disconcerting. The potential to improve medical care through more effective use of our knowledge is considerable, but the potential for misuse, and the fear for the doctor–patient relationship, was worrying. No profession readily accepts that its position can be usurped by a machine.

After the initial enthusiasm and confidence, doubt has set in. Much has been achieved, but the high hopes have not been realized, and some believe that they never will be. No doubt many doctors will be relieved to hear this, but for anyone interested in reducing uncertainty in medicine, this is a disappointment. So, what is the problem and exactly what has been achieved?

The problem lies in the difficulty of programming the more imaginative aspects of human thinking into a computer. This may, in part, be because we do not understand this aspect of thinking, and workers in the field of artificial intelligence have realized that we need to know more about the thinking process before further advances can be made. This has led to the relatively recent development of the field of cognitive science, but the truth is that philosophers have argued over these problems for centuries. Some of these arguments have been discussed in Chapter 2 of this book, and before discussing the various types of computer systems available to aid diagnosis, it is useful to extend the philosophy a little further. The basic question is how do we think, and how far can a computer simulate these processes. In short, can a computer think?

CAN A COMPUTER THINK?

The computer resembles the human brain in many respects, so it would not be unreasonable to expect computers to produce similar results. A computer works by processing a series of pulses which are all or nothing events like nerve impulses. These pulses can be processed by addition and subtraction, simple processes which when used on a large scale in a sophisticated way can produce complex results. Individual neurones can serve the same function. Transmission of pulses in computer circuits is far faster than along neurones, and the processing is also quicker. So why is it that the tortoise outruns the hare?

The essential difference may be that nervous systems are parallel machines with signals being processed in millions of neurones simultaneously instead of in sequence as in the computer. Whilst it is possible to produce computer systems with parallel processing, this development is still rudimentary. Computing through parallel circuits has three major advantages:

1. Since processing can occur in many areas of the neural network simultaneously there are clear advantages in the speed of computation.

2. There is also the advantage that information is distributed widely throughout the network in the form of differences in synaptic resistance due to the previous passage of impulses. In effect this memory is stored as molecular changes at nerve endings which can directly influence the computation. There is even evidence that the synaptic connections themselves can become disconnected and reconnected. By these means the hardware can be continually updated.

3. A further advantage is the in-built redundancy possible with parallel circuits which ensures that the loss of a few neurones has negligible effect on the overall function of the brain. Naturally, there is a limit as to how many neurones can be removed before function deteriorates, but it is remarkable how much of the brain can be affected by diffuse pathological processes such as cerebral ischaemia before serious problems develop. In this respect the brain resembles a holographic picture in which the picture is still apparent in its entirety even when a section is cut out, only the definition is reduced.

Most people consider humans to be more effective than machines because we are conscious and able to think. To such people the idea that machines may think carries little credence, yet the basic neurophysiological processes in the brain and computer electronics show similarities, and whilst current computers are relatively simple by comparison, there seems to be no fundamental reason why future hardware should not match the brain. Most people accept that the physical brain is responsible for consciousness, so why should the computer not be conscious and able to think? If computers can think, there is every reason to expect that in the course of time computer decision making will have a significant role to play in medical care.

The question has been hotly debated; there are those who believe that computers cannot think and probably never will be able to, but there are those who are equally adamant that they can. When asked if machines think, Claude Shannon, the father of information theory, answered in unequivocal terms, 'You bet. We're machines and we think, don't we?' There are others who have given a more analytical answer; anyone interested in this debate should read the contrasting views in the *Scientific American* (January, 1990).

The people best known for their doubts about the potential sophistication of computer systems are John Searle and Hubert Dreyfus, both professors of philosophy at the University of California, and Stuart Dreyfus who is a professor of industrial engineering. Their conclusions are the same, but their arguments differ.

John Searle argues that syntax is not sufficient for semantics. The moving around of symbols—syntax—is not sufficient to explain the understanding of the meaning of words and situations—semantics—which seems crucial to human thinking. This Searle accepts as a basic axiom, and since computer systems are purely syntactic it follows that computers cannot think.

He uses the analogy of the Chinese room in which a man sits with access to a comprehensive set of rules for manipulating Chinese symbols. The rule book is written in English, and the man does not understand Chinese. Whenever a question containing a set of Chinese characters is pushed into his room, he consults the rules, chooses the appropriate Chinese characters from numbered bins, and the answer is posted back. If the rules are comprehensive the correct answer will have been given to the question. The crucial point is that the man has no idea, no mental image, of what the question was, and has no idea of the answer he has given. He does not understand the meaning of the symbols—semantics—but juggling with the order of the symbols—syntax—leads him to give the correct answer because the rules are correct. In other words, the man is acting like the central processor of a computer.

The difficulty is that not everyone accepts the axiom that syntax is insufficient for semantics. Some say that the juggling of syntactic elements can produce the same cognitive states to those found in humans. Supporters of what has been called strong artificial intelligence believe that if a computer can simulate thinking in such a way that an expert cannot distinguish between its performance and that of a human, then a computer has the ability to think. There seems to be no other way of deciding whether a computer can think or not except on the basis of how a computer behaves and how it interacts with us. This forms the basis of the Turing test which derives from the principles laid down by Alan Turing in 1950 in his influential paper, 'Computing machinery and intelligence'.[56] In that computers do not quite behave like humans, with our irrational thoughts and intuitive behaviour, it is easy to think that we are essentially different, but this may be due to deficiencies in our current level of technology. Anyone interested in the detailed arguments concerning the Turing principle should read Roger Penrose's book *The Emperor's New Mind*.[57]

Hubert and Stuart Dreyfus[44] approached the problem by studying the cognitive process. The question is the degree to which thinking is based on application of rules, which computers are eminently suited to deal with, in a rational deductive process as previously described in Chapter 2 and attributed to Descartes. Kant (1724–1804) had based his philosophy on the assumption that all concepts were rule-based, of the form, 'A dog is a dog because it has four legs, barks and wags its tail'; and Husserl (1859–1938) extended this further with his concept of hierarchies of rules which describe phenomena at different levels of precision. Whilst it has not yet proved possible to build up a full description of the world from basic axioms and a set of rules, these rational philosophers would see no fundamental reason why this should not eventually be achieved.

This view has not gone unchallenged. Pascal (1623–62), who was himself a mathematician, argued that we do not have access to universal axioms which are beyond dispute. We base our ideas on knowledge gained from custom and experience. As he put it, 'The heart has its reasons that reason does not know'.

Our understanding of the world has to be based on our everyday experience. Heidegger (1889–1976), Wittgenstein (1889–1951), and Merleau-Ponty (1908–61) concluded that perception could not be explained by the application of rules. We need to know how to find our way around the world. It is not sufficient to know a lot of facts and rules relating them; it is the knowing how, rather than the knowing that, which is important. Rules are best when not treated rigidly, and should be seen in the context of a flexible style of behaviour. We could, for example, define a set of rules concerning the meaning and function of a stick. It could be described as a support for plants, but we could find many different functions for a stick apart from this; some readers may even have discovered one as an errant schoolchild. Even a monkey will use a stick for gathering food from outside his cage. We could extend the set of rules to cover as many functions as we know, but what sets man and higher animals apart from machines is that other possible uses can be imagined.

Favouring these non-rational philosophers, Hubert Dreyfus had doubts about the ability of a computer system to rival the brain. His brother developed similar doubts and, after explaining his work in computer decision making to an acquaintance at a social gathering, he gave his favourite example of how a computer could be used to guide one in the purchase of a car. You estimate the cost of a new car, etc., and the computer makes the decision. On this occasion someone asked him, 'Is this the way you decide how to replace your car?' The obvious quick answer to this was, 'Of course not, I buy a new car when it feels right.' What was different about the human decision making process?

The difference is that computers lack the intuition, inspiration and insight which the brain uses in coming to decisions. Computer systems, by contrast, work on a purely rational basis. As we saw in Chapters 2 and 3, the rational processes of deduction and hypothetico-deductive reasoning are important ways of thinking which can be used with great benefit. With experience, though, experts increasingly use intuitive methods even though they might have to revert to hypothetico-deductive methods for unfamiliar problems. In their book, *Mind over Machine*,[44] Hubert and Stuart Dreyfus define five steps in the evolution of expert thinking which we touched upon in Chapter 3 under the heading of 'The Cognitive Continuum'. Further details can be found in their book, but the reader will probably appreciate that decisions are made by intuitive methods increasingly as experience is gained. Anyone who drives a car will realize that an inexperienced driver drives by consciously obeying the rules, not the rules of the road, although it is hoped that they do so, but the rules of the driving process itself. As experience is gained, the driver becomes less conscious of the rules and decisions made. The car becomes an extension of the body and the driver can respond appropriately to situations, even those he has not experienced before.

Anyone familiar with the television series, *Star Trek*, will recognize the difference between highly rational thought, demonstrated by computers and Mr Spock, and intuitive thought, so important in making decisions based on uncertainty. Whilst Mr Spock was an invaluable member of the crew, when the chips were down it was Captain James Kirk who did the right thing, often for what seemed to be the wrong reason. He epitomizes human irrational thought so alien to Mr Spock.

Whether computers can think or not, it is clear that, at the moment, computers do not work in an intuitive manner. There is nothing to suggest from their behaviour that they conceptualize a problem as formal conscious images. True, they can manipulate images, but even this facility is limited. Nor can computers exhibit the properties of common-sense thought; despite work on the common-sense knowledge approach to computing it has not been possible to reproduce the common-sense understanding of a four year old. Whether these weaknesses are due to intrinsic flaws in computer methodology, or whether it is due to computer systems still being in their infancy, is difficult to say. But whatever the reason, and even with the modern cognitive models used in decision analysis, we are still a long way from emulating the thinking process of the expert.

THE DEVELOPMENT OF COMPUTER ASSISTED DIAGNOSIS

The partitioning of a continuous process into different historical epochs is bound to be a questionable over-simplification, but the exercise does help to emphasize the direction in which experts in the field are travelling. As far as computer assisted diagnosis is concerned, the first systems, developed in the 1960s, used an algorithmic approach for which the computer is particularly well suited. This decade can be considered as the algorithmic period and, despite being the first systems developed, in many respects algorithmic systems are still as useful as the more modern programs. They are, however, relatively rigid systems more suited to well defined and limited problems.

This period overlapped with the era in which computer programs were based on the statistical approach. As with algorithmic methods there was no intention at this time to simulate the thinking process, but merely to develop a useable system which was at least as accurate as a physician. As long as this could be achieved there was no particular advantage in copying the human mind.

When there is no obvious causal connection between events, there is no particular advantage to be gained in using any other system. However, in other circumstances, there are potential advantages in developing systems which can behave rationally using deductive processes. This led to the development of systems which use rules in much the same way that humans use the deductive process. Given a knowledge base, and a set of rules, systems can be developed to deduce, in the Cartesian sense, necessary consequences which in this case are diagnoses. In that these production rule systems are beginning to exhibit characteristics similar to human intelligence, this era can be considered as the birth of artificial intelligence.

The next phase was the development of cognitive models which simulate the hypothesis and test approach of the hypothetico-deductive method. To a certain extent this can be achieved with production rule systems using the top-down approach which will be looked at later, but the cognitive models are far more sophisticated. One of the main strengths of this approach is that the knowledge base is held in frames of associated information which makes it much more practical to develop. The system can be developed in units and function with increasingly wide applications as more units are added.

The modern era may see the further development of more general software systems which simulate the thinking process and to which different databases can be added. Such systems would have the advantage of allowing local databases to be used. There may also be an increasing move towards diagnostic prompting systems in which the user is intermittently involved in the diagnostic process, but with the computer helping at points in the diagnostic process which are proving difficult. These systems have the combined advantage of a large database as well as expert thinking provided by the physician, and are not dissimilar from using the computer like a consultant's opinion.

Computer aided diagnostic systems raise exciting possibilities, not so much for the majority of patients in whom diagnosis presents no great problem, but in terms of their potential help in difficult cases. With the increasing sophistication of computer hardware and networks, one can imagine smaller hospitals having access to computer systems based in larger centres. A younger generation of doctors brought up in the computer era is unlikely to feel intimidated by such possibilities.

The types of systems currently available will now be reviewed in brief. Anyone interested in a further description of this field should refer to *Computers and Medicine: Computer Assisted Medical Decision Making* (Volumes 1 and 2), edited by Reggia and Tuhrim,[58] who provide an excellent introductory chapter where an extensive bibliography can be found. The reader may be confused by the interchange between the terms artificial intelligence and expert systems. Different people seem to use the terms in different ways. One definition of artifical intelligence is that it is a system which simulates human intelligence and learns, whilst an expert system does not have the facility for learning new rules or changing the database. At other times the term expert system is used to describe systems in which the knowledge of experts, in this case doctors, has been used for the database and collection of rules.

ALGORITHMIC SYSTEMS

Algorithms are logical systems introduced by the Arabian mathematician Al-Khwarizmi (9th century AD). They are based on a series of IF . . . THEN statements which lend themselves to computer programming. The use of algorithms is not limited to computer systems, and most doctors will have seen algorithmic trees which can be used for diagnostic problems. There are several publications of such algorithms for use in medicine, and they can undoubtedly be useful, particularly in highly specialized areas. Their great advantage is that they give a consistent answer, and can be used by non-experts. In effect, they are written by experts for use by non-experts. One of the disadvantages, though, is that an adequate algorithm can be unwieldy. Taken step by step they are simple to use, but seen in their entirety they can certainly appear formidable and offputting, although having the algorithm written as a program in a computer makes them more user-friendly.

A very simple algorithm is shown in Figure 5.1, and, whilst this is too simplified to be of any practical use, it does

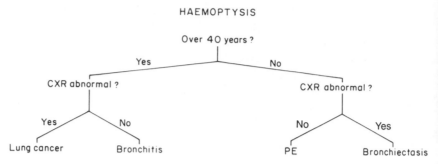

Figure 5.1   *Clinical algorithm for haemoptysis. CXR: chest X-ray; PE: pulmonary embolism.*

demonstrate the idea and shows some of the limitations. Algorithms can be written in different forms, but in essence they ask questions to which there is a yes/no answer. The logic part of it is in the IF . . . THEN statements. For example, in the figure shown, if a patient is over 40 and has a chest X-ray abnormality then the patient has lung cancer. Clearly this algorithm is absurdly over-simplified, but even more sophisticated algorithms tend to be logically over-simplistic. It is virtually impossible to cover all eventualities, and the required yes/no answer is often not possible. Algorithms do not cater for uncertainty and they rely on accurate observation at all times.

Nevertheless, successful algorithms have been developed some of which have been incorporated into computer systems. They have been particularly successful in the evaluation of a patient's acid base status[59] and in the determination of drug dosages[60] taking into account the patient's age, sex, weight, previous drug dosage as well as the pharmacokinetics of the drug. Algorithms are best drawn up with a view to minimizing path length with clear objectives in mind and with the most discriminating questions asked at each node. Undoubtedly they have a role to play in the medical decision making process, but their use without computer aids can be tedious and time consuming. Even with the help of computers their lack of flexibility limits their usefulness.

STATISTICAL SYSTEMS

Some of the most successful systems developed have been based on a statistical approach to problem solving. Central to these methods is the acceptance of uncertainty as a problem intrinsic to the diagnostic process. The diagnosis is not made on the basis of pathophysiological reasoning and causality, but on the statistical relationship between clinical findings and potential diagnosis. This carries an inherent disadvantage, namely the lack of a diagnosis reasoned in the understandable pathophysiological terms which doctors like to see. Many people find it difficult to empathize with this numerical approach.

Most systems use the concepts of Bayesian statistics discussed in Chapter 4, and some use the method of linear discriminant functions which is a variant of this type of statistics. The knowledge base consists of information in the form of $P(F|D)$, and the weaknesses inherent in this approach apply just as much to these computer systems.

Nevertheless, one of the most successful systems introduced is a Bayesian system which can be applied to patients with abdominal pain.[61] This has been one of the most thoroughly evaluated systems involving 16 737 patients and over 250 doctors.[62] It improved the accuracy of initial diagnosis from 45% to 65% and the post-investigation diagnostic accuracy from 58% to 74%. The negative laparotomy rate fell by almost a half and the observed mortality by 22%. This increased accuracy led to substantial financial savings. Interestingly, approximately half of this improvement was due to the more structured data collection necessary for the computer system which could be introduced relatively cheaply and more cost-effectively than the computer technology.

A different statistical approach is the use of database comparisons. This entails collection of a large database containing the salient features about patients which are relevant to the diagnosis. The clinical features of a new patient are then compared with this database and the best comparison found. It is unlikely that the new patient will have identical features to a patient in the database, and this method is classified as statistical because the match is based on the nearest rather than a perfect fit. Systems using this technique have been developed particularly for prognostic expectations, but also to aid in the diagnostic process.

One major disadvantage is that this approach requires a large database before it can usefully function; this database is best collected from the practice of the user. This puts heavy demands on the available resources, let alone on the computer hardware. The system is inefficient in terms of computer memory and processing time. It also relies on careful identification of the important features, which should be independent and strongly correlated with prognosis.

One major advantage compared with Bayesian systems is that no assumption is made about the independence of clinical features. The database consists of hard evidence rather than estimates of prior probability and conditional probabilities. Collection of such data through medical audit is in tune with modern trends and data collected can be used in Bayesian systems which allow the database to be tailed for local application.

PRODUCTION RULE SYSTEMS

This type of system falls into the category of artificial intelligence because it simulates one of the ways the human mind can think, namely using rational, deductive processes. It is based on a set of conditional rules of the form

IF (antecedent) . . . THEN (consequences)

and in this regard there are similarities with the algorithmic system. But this type of system differs in that the set of production rules need not be used in any fixed pattern. Indeed, not all rules will be needed for the diagnosis of a particular patient. Furthermore, more rules can be added, although this is not always straightforward because of the possibility of interaction between rules. An important part of the program—called a rule interpreter—selects the rules to use for a particular case.

There are a number of variations of this basic approach in use. Some use a purely deductive logic in antecedent driven fashion (bottom up). Others state the consequence first, and check if the necessary facts, the antecedents, are found in the details of that particular patient. The consequence driven, top-down, or backward chaining, approach is similar to the hypothetico-deductive method with the hypothesis being stated first, and the consequence of this hypothesis then being evaluated. Rules may be chained together to make multiple step deductions, and it is possible to state consequences in terms of less than absolute certainty which can then be propagated from one rule to the next using numerical methods.

A major problem with this approach follows from the difficulty in laying down hard and fast rules in medicine, which is not solely due to difficulties in liaison between expert doctors and computer scientists. We have seen that doctors, particularly expert doctors, often do not make diagnoses according to set rules, preferring to use the intuitive approach. This is not new. Plato related an encounter between Socrates and Euthyphro when Socrates asked Euthyphro for the rules on identifying piety. Euthyphro did what others tended to do when cornered by Socrates and gave him examples from his experience. Socrates persisted in asking for the rules, but although Euthyphro claimed to know how to tell pious acts from non-pious acts, he could not lay down any rules. Socrates had no more joy out of craftsmen, poets and statesmen on making enquiries into their fields of interest, and he concluded that no-one knew anything!

The logical problems of the modern era are no different from those of ancient Greece, but to return to the specific weaknesses of production rule systems, one further problem is that many findings in medicine are context-dependent. The significance of lumbar pain depends on other features such as associated sciatica, foot drop, urinary retention, known cancer, etc. Whilst it is possible to define lumbar pain with any or all of these features in separate antecedent clauses, the number of production rules generated can rise rapidly.

Rule based systems have been developed for several areas of medicine including the choice of antibacterial drugs for infection (MYSIN),[63] and the diagnosis and treatment of glaucoma (CASNET/Glaucoma)[64] as well as in the interpretation of pulmonary function tests (PUFF).[65] One advantage that these systems do have over statistical systems is a limited explanatory function. At the very least the production rules used to come to a diagnosis can be made available to the user, but the major difficulty of stating precise production rules is an intrinsic limitation which cannot be easily overcome.

COGNITIVE MODELS

Systems falling into this category, which are based more closely on the normal thinking processes of man, are still in their infancy and present formidable programming challenges. They are based on the hypothetico-deductive mode of reasoning. The database is held in frames of associated knowledge. Each pivotal feature, sometimes known as a 'problem knowledge coupler',[66] has a frame of relevant knowledge which can be brought into short-term memory and explored when the computer is triggered by the appropriate input. Other frames, containing relevant but less closely associated information, may be drawn near a short-term memory, but not necessarily explored. A set of possible hypotheses are then generated and tested by various scoring procedures which measure the ability to account for the known clinical findings.

Some systems use production rules as well as these concepts, but in most cases the diagnostic knowledge is described in a form more familiar to doctors and so helps the user to interrelate with the system. A further advantage is that the modular construction of the program, with information being held in frames, allows the system to be developed in stages. Initially, the program may have a limited application, but as more frames are added the application of the system widens. Examples of such systems developed include one for general medicine (INTERNIST I)[67] as well as cholestasis (MDX)[68] and neurology (NEUROLOGIST).[69]

Whilst the development of these systems presents formidable programming challenges, they do offer great promise. However, there is one problem which will not be easy to overcome and that is the difficulty of dealing with multiple simultaneous diagnoses. It is possible for the program to get hold of the wrong end of the stick and begin with analysis of inappropriate aspects of the case. This is not, of course, unfamiliar to the human diagnostician, but an attribute of experts is that they are good at avoiding this. How this is achieved remains unclear and so makes it impossible to assimilate in a computer.

A number of possible solutions to this problem have been suggested, perhaps the most encouraging being the formulation of a theoretical foundation for cognitive systems. Statistical systems are based on probability theory and rule based systems are based on first order predicate calculus. The mathematical model of generalized set covering has been suggested as a basis for cognitive systems. The clinical features of the case have to be explained, and the minimal set of diseases which can adequately cover all these manifestations can be found using the principles of this method.

PERFORMANCE ASSESSMENT

Evaluation of computer aided diagnostic systems is difficult, and there are few examples in the literature of adequate comparisons with physicians' opinions, although the paper by Adams et al.[62] is a notable exception to this. One of the difficulties is in defining unequivocally what the correct diagnosis is. Ideally a prospective clinical evaluation is desirable in which the final diagnosis is likely to be certain, but this would be difficult to implement. A computer system could be compared with an expert, for example, in the diagnosis of appendicitis, but accuracy could only be assessed by knowing for certain whether a patient did or did not have appendicitis, and this might entail performing appendicectomies even in those patients diagnosed as not having appendicitis. The independent gold standard would then be the pathologist's report, but ethical objections would make it impossible to mount such a study.

A more realistic, but less satisfactory approach, is to measure the agreement between computer systems and experts. If agreement is good at least one can say that the system is as good as an expert and, by implication, better than a non-expert. The problem is similar to that described previously when the agreement between different physicians about clinical findings was discussed. Chance agreement has to be taken into consideration, and this can be achieved using the statistic kappa (x);

$$kappa = \frac{P_o - P_c}{1 - P_c}$$

where P_o is the observed agreement, and P_c the agreement which can be attributed to chance.

The relationship can be seen best by marking the agreement rates on a line.

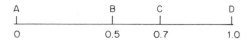

where C = observed agreement rate and B = the chance agreement rate of 0.5 (chosen arbitrarily for this particular example).

$$kappa = \frac{C-B}{D-B} = 0.4$$

i.e. only 40% of the potential improvement in agreement is achieved; the observed agreement rate of 70% can be seen to be misleading. Using this statistic, a value of x equal to 1.0 indicates perfect agreement, and x equal to 0 occurs when there is pure chance agreement.

A further problem in assessing performance is that a comparison of this type does not take into account the probabilistic nature of making a diagnosis. A computer diagnosis which gives a correct diagnosis, but only with a probability of 0.55, would get the same 'marks' as a system which gives the same diagnosis, but with a probability of 0.95. Measuring accuracy without taking this into account loses important information. A statistical method using accuracy coefficients can be used to give a better assessment in this type of situation.

There are, therefore, limitations in our ability to assess the performance of computer systems although, by and large, this would also apply to comparing the performance of physicians. What studies have shown is that computer systems can be as good as physicians, and even better in some circumstances.[62] There have also been comparisons between computers, with machine being pitted against machine. It is natural to ask what is the best type of system, but the better question to ask is which system is more suitable to the type of problem to which it is to be applied. This will depend on the form in which the knowledge is held. If the information available is present in statistical terms, with poor understanding of the causal relationships between findings and diagnosis, then a statistical based system is more appropriate. A Bayesian system would be preferred if the clinical features measured are mutually independent, and the conditional probabilities known. On the other hand, if our understanding of the problem can be stated in well defined rules, then rule based systems might be more appropriate. This would be particularly true if the findings are not strongly context dependent. A cognitive system might be more appropriate when the knowledge base is mainly descriptive, and there is a mixture of probabilistic and causal relationships involved. This is the common situation in general medical applications where cognitive systems are more promising. A rule based system may be more appropriate for management of a patient whose diagnosis has already been established, and Bayesian systems more appropriate for medical problems with limited input information.

PROBLEMS IN THE APPLICATION OF COMPUTER DIAGNOSTIC SYSTEMS

As with Bayesian statistics and decision analysis, it is not unreasonable to ask why it is that computer systems are not in general use if they are such a good thing. It is true to say that they have not yet lived up to their initial promise in terms of accuracy, but some systems have been shown to be at least as good as experts.

One of the problems is that they would have to be shown to be better than experts if they are to justify their expense. The expense is not simply the cost of hardware and software, but, more importantly, there is the question of time. Making a computer diagnosis can be a slow process by the time the computer is accessed, data put in, and the interaction with the physician, if needed, is complete. Clearly, the computer would only be used in cases where diagnostic difficulties arise, but in these circumstances time spent in the library or discussing the case with colleagues may achieve the same end. The difficulty may be in finding the time, rather than any weakness of knowledge base or inference mechanism.

One of the limitations intrinsic to the method is that it is unlikely that a computer will be better than the expert who provides the knowledge base and rules. True, it can be made as good as the expert on a good day with time to think, but this is nevertheless a significant limitation. Problems in making a diagnosis may be due to inaccuracy of findings and paucity of understanding rather than weaknesses in inference. Statistical systems suffer from a lack of reliable information about conditional probability, and the prior probability of disease, which is crucial to the final likelihood of a diagnosis, may not be known for the local population. The system may, therefore, not be readily transferable from one centre to another.

A key element in expert performance, which is difficult to simulate in a computer, is the physician's ability to limit the number of hypotheses under consideration at any one time. It was mentioned in Chapter 3 that physicians seldom hold more than four possible causes of illness in their minds simultaneously, and this can be advantageous. The whole process of diagnosis is one of narrowing the options, and yet computer systems can lead to an explosion of possible hypotheses.

With a number of clinical features characterizing a clinical problem the computer could be programmed to choose possible diagnoses using a Boolean AND, or a Boolean OR, function. For anyone unfamiliar with Boolean algebra, the Boolean AND function would lead to the computer printing out only diagnoses that would explain all the clinical features. For example, a patient with gastroenteritis may have vomiting, diarrhoea and fever; using a Boolean AND function, all these features would have to be present for the diagnosis to be made. But every practising physician knows that patients rarely have all the features of a disease, so the choice of a Boolean AND function would lead to premature exclusion of real possibilities, although it would avoid an explosion in the number of possible diagnoses. On the other hand, the Boolean OR function would have the opposite effect. Any diagnosis which could explain any one of the features would have to be considered, and in this particular example this would mean that all cases of vomiting, diarrhoea or fever would have to be considered as possible causes of the patient's illness. This avoids premature exclusion, but generates a long list of possible diagnoses, although the situation can be improved by ranking the hypotheses according to how many of the clinical features can be explained by each diagnosis.

Where the computer is weak, the physician can help. By choosing and identifying the pivotal features of the case, the physician is able to ensure that the computer restricts its search to a more relevant field. Deactivation of the hypothesis when it fails to account for a significant proportion of pivotal features is also important, but it could be relegated to a catch-all category which could then be explored if the favoured hypothesis proves untenable. The aggregation of hypotheses into similar groups such as vasculitic disorders can also simplify the job of the computer. The usefulness of these techniques to narrow the field of possible diagnoses should not be surprising since they are used by the practising physician.

A further difficulty is that the innate conservatism which is endemic in the medical profession, particularly towards anything which seems to threaten the doctor/patient relationship, presents a problem in acceptance. There is a reluctance to rely on a computer aid in making a diagnosis which is in marked contrast to the ready acceptance of a new diagnostic test. It is only right to question whether an innovation is needed and whether it really improves performance. This is true of any innovation in medicine, but doctors do not always apply the same strict rules to other developments.

Another general point is the real risk of successful computer systems taking the intellectual challenge out of medicine thus leading to lack of interest. Physicians prefer the type of system with which they can interact, or at least follow the reasoning which has led to the diagnosis and, fortunately, there is a move in that direction. Although it has proved difficult to program the pathophysiological reasoning which is so important in the physician's diagnostic process, it has proved possible to store a set of causal associations which can be used to justify a decision even when these are not used directly in problem solving. Research workers see this 'answer justification' as a key research goal for the future. Perhaps the future may also see the development of more advanced technology for interfacing with the computer; the use of 19th century technology, the keyboard, is offputting to those who are not expert typists.

As to the fear of some physicians about the concept of a computer making life and death decisions, they should bear in mind that computers fly aeroplanes and run underground train networks. The physician should take comfort from the fact that he will always be needed to provide the ultimate safety of a well developed intuitive mind.

FURTHER READING

Chard, T. *Computing for Clinicians*. London: Elmore—Chard, 1988.

Churchland, P. M., Churchland, P. S. and Searle, J. R. Artificial intelligence: a debate. *Scientific American* 1990; Jan: 20–31.

Dreyfus, H. L. and Dreyfus, S. E. *Mind over Machine*. Oxford: Blackwell, 1986.

Pollock, R. V. H. Diagnosis by calculation. *Compendium of Continuing Education for the Practicing Veterinarian* 1985; 7: 1019–1034.

Reggia, J. A. and Tuhrim, S. (eds.) *Computers and Medicine: Computer Assisted Decision Making*, Vol. 1 and 2. New York: Springer Verlag, 1985.

Szdovits, P., Patil, R. S. and Schwarz, W. B. Artificial intelligence in medical diagnosis. *Annals of Internal Medicine* 1988; **108**: 80–87.

6
Decision Analysis

'Errors of judgement must occur in the practice of an art which consists largely in balancing probabilities.'

Osler

INTRODUCTION

So far attention has been focused on difficulties encountered in the definition and diagnosis of disease, but even when the diagnosis is clear the best management option may still be uncertain. In this chapter, the emphasis changes from the problems of making a diagnosis, to problems of dealing with the uncertainty involved in managing illness. One kind of treatment may have a high cure rate, and yet a small percentage of patients may be worse or even die because of the treatment. With the same clinical problem another type of treatment may have only a low cure rate, but may be much safer. What is the best option to choose?

Anyone who doubts the existence of wide variations in medical practice—and there can be few practising doctors to whom this could apply—need only glance at the literature to convince themselves that inconsistencies abound. This was convincingly shown in a study which looked at the advice given to schoolchildren with recurrent tonsillitis (Figure 6.1).[70] At the time the study was published, tonsillectomy was a popular approach to this problem and out of 1000 children with this problem a group of doctors decided that 611 required tonsillectomy. The 389 children for whom tonsillectomy was not advised were taken

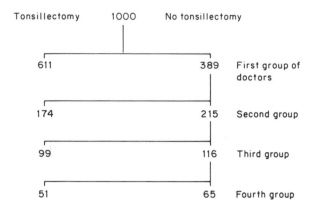

Figure 6.1 *Decisions of four groups of doctors as to whether tonsillectomy should be advised for 1000 children with recurrent throat infections.*

to a second group of doctors and the same question with regard to tonsillectomy was asked. It was now decided that 174 of these children required tonsillectomy after all. Undaunted by this finding the authors had a third opinion on the remaining 215 children to discover that 99 of them required surgery. The reader will not be surprised to discover that the intrepid research workers took the remaining 116 to yet another group of doctors and that they advised 51 to have surgery. Out of the original 1000 children only 65 had been consistently advised not to have tonsillectomy. At that point they ran out of doctors!

Whenever more than one management option exists there are likely to be different risks and advantages to each approach making the option finally chosen a gamble. There are, however, techniques belonging to the field of decision analysis which can at least optimize the outcome when the options and outcomes desired are clearly defined; but it always follows, when dealing with uncertainty, that correct decisions can have bad outcomes in the same way that bad decisions, by chance, may have good outcomes. Even when formal methods of decision analysis are applied, the decision remains a gamble, and it is a gamble that is usually taken by the doctor on behalf of his patient. Alternatively, techniques based on gambling theory are available which allow patients to participate fully in decisions about their health. In this chapter the basic concepts of formal decision analysis will be explored using simple examples, but we shall also look at the very real limitations of applying formal techniques to the diagnosis and management of medical problems.

There are three steps involved in making a formal decision analysis.

1. *The formulation of a decision tree.* This summarizes the options available and possible outcomes. To be useful it has to be relatively simple but also realistic. The decision tree in Figure 6.2 shows the two types of branching available: a decision node, the symbol for which is a box, is a point in the decision tree at which a choice has to be made. A chance node, the symbol for which is a circle, is a point at which chance dictates the outcome. Creating the decision tree is the most difficult part of the exercise, but is an excellent opportunity to clarify the problem. Some people have argued against formal decision analysis on the basis that it takes the art out of medicine, but considerable art is involved in making a satisfactory decision tree.

2. *The desired outcomes must be defined.* In a simple analysis, this would be to maximize the average life expectancy if a particular

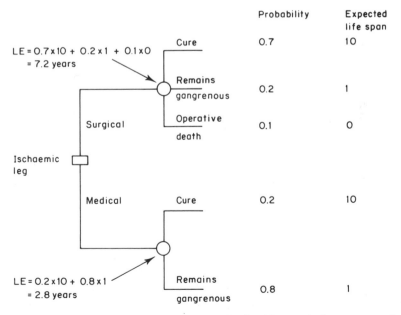

Figure 6.2 *Decision tree comparing medical with surgical treatment for ischaemic legs.*

decision, or series of decisions, are taken. Alternatively, the outcome sought could be the life expectancy adjusted for the quality of life, the best combination of outcome and cost (cost effectiveness), or some other desired outcome such as minimum discomfort. When the patient is directly involved in making the decisions, the strength of a patient's preference for an outcome is known as the utility.
3. *The decision tree is then folded back.* The expected value of each decision has to be calculated in terms of life expectancy, cost, utility or whatever outcome variable has been chosen. This process is known as folding back the decision tree, and consists of calculating the average effect of a decision taking into account the various potential outcomes and the possibility of each one of these occurring.

A few examples will now be given to explore the methods in more detail. They are deliberately chosen to be simple and some are based on the excellent book on medical decision making by Sox et al.[71] but the values quoted should not be regarded as based on accurate information. There are many published papers in which these techniques have been used and the interested reader might like to refer to the paper published by Kassirer et al.[72] which contains a progress report to 1987 with numerous references.

LIFE EXPECTANCY ANALYSIS

Consider the decision which has to be made about a diabetic patient who has an ischaemic leg. The two principal options are to treat this medically or to treat surgically by amputation. Naturally, the actual options are more extensive than this. For example, one would be to treat medically for a few more weeks and then intervene with surgery if progress is not satisfactory. This could be included in the analysis, but my aim is to generate a very simple decision tree for clarity.

Figure 6.2 shows the decision tree from which it can be seen that the decision node is between surgery or medical treatment. If the surgical option is taken, there are three possible outcomes at the chance node: i.e. cure, stump gangrene or operative death.

Immediate or early death is not likely with medical treatment, so the two outcome options with medical treatment are for the leg to remain gangrenous, or cure.

Having drawn up the decision tree, the next step is to assign the likelihood of each possible outcome. These figures should be available from the literature or the personal experience of the doctor making the decision. As will be discussed later, one of the weaknesses of formal decision analysis is the scarcity of accurate data from which such probabilities can be derived. The expected life span for each of these outcomes should now be found. Once again, data from the literature or personal experience will be important in deciding this for a person who has a gangrenous limb. The expected life span of a person who is cured depends upon his age and the detrimental effect of the underlying problem—in this case, diabetes. We shall come back to the calculation of this, but for the moment let us accept the figure of 10 years.

All that remains to be done now is to calculate the average life expectancy at the chance node. This is the sum of the product of probability times life expectancy for each outcome as shown in Figure 6.2. The average life expectancy of 7.2 years for surgical treatment is clearly better than the average life expectancy for medical treatment. The best overall decision would be surgical treatment, even though there is a risk of early death due to the operation.

With more complicated decision trees, there may be two or more chance nodes in series in which case the life expectancy for the first, most peripheral branch, is used as the starting point for the second branch. Similarly, there may well be more than one decision node, and the branch with the highest expected value is chosen to continue the folding back procedure, the other branches being ignored. In effect, the decision tree becomes progressively simplified as the calculations proceed towards the main trunk of the tree. This is what is meant by folding back the decision tree.

Life expectancy is an important and easily understood endpoint for evaluating treatment. It may seem less than spectacular if a patient only lives for 10 years after an operation, but if the patient is aged 70 at the time of the operation the likelihood is that the patient will die from some other cause. Clearly the age

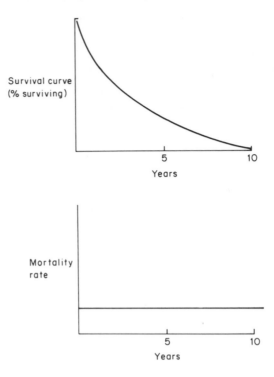

Figure 6.3   *Basis of the DEALE method for calculating life expectancy.*

of the patient is an important factor in life expectancy, and so also is the presence of any other disease. The simplest way of calculating life expectancy is to assume a declining exponential approximation of life expectancy—DEALE.[73] This assumes a constant mortality rate, but any error incurred by this assumption is small except when applied to a particularly young person. The mortality rate is derived from data available in the literature about survival after the onset of an illness or after a procedure (Figure 6.3). The basic assumption of the method is that the following reciprocal relationship between life expectancy (LE) and mortality rate holds:

$$LE = \frac{1}{M}$$

and M, the mortality rate, is related to survival by the exponential function

$$S = S_0 \cdot e^{-Mt}$$

or

$$M = (-1/t) \cdot \ln(S/S_0)$$

where S = number of patients surviving at time t, S_0 = number of patients alive at time 0, t = time at which fractional survival is measured.

These three measurements—S, S_0, and t—are relatively easily obtained and form the basic data from which mortality figures are derived.

Total mortality rate consists of mortality specific to the disease in question and mortality related to the age of the patient, which is the sum of mortality due to all other causes. The relationship is given by:

$$M_{total} = M_{disease\ specific} + M_{age\ specific}$$

To calculate life expectancy for the decision tree you need to know the disease specific mortality for the illness or procedure in question, which is obtained from the literature, and the age specific mortality, for a patient of that particular age, obtained from the appropriate life tables. If more than one disease is present then

$$M_{total} = M_{age\ specific} + M_{disease\ 1} + M_{disease\ 2}$$

as long as the two diseases do not interact.

There are a number of assumptions made with this method, apart from the reciprocal relationship between life expectancy and mortality, but the method works well with the majority of cases and is much simpler than alternatives such as the Gompertz function and Markov Process. An outline of alternative ways of calculating life expectancy is given in *Medical Decision Analysis* by Sox et al.[71] where the accuracy of the DEALE method is discussed further.

QUALITY ADJUSTED LIFE YEAR—QALY

Anyone who has looked after patients in pain or suffering disability will have quickly realized that the length of life is not all that needs to be considered when making a medical decision; quality of life is also of paramount importance and this can be incorporated into decision analysis using the concept of a quality adjusted life year—QALY.[74] This is defined as a period of time in perfect health that a patient regards as equivalent to a year in a state of ill health. A patient with angina, for example, may have a life expectancy of 12 years, but would be willing to accept a life expectancy of 9 years if only he could be cured of his angina. In the language of decision analysis his expected life span is equivalent to 9 QALYs. The fundamental principle of a QALY, therefore, is that it combines quality of life with length of life in one value which can then be used for comparative purposes.

Consider the patient with intermittent claudication who faces the choice of an operation with a good chance of cure, but with a small chance of death. This has to be compared with medical treatment with only partial suppression of symptoms. To complicate matters further, there is a small chance that even if the patient survives the operation the problem will not be cured. Figure 6.4 shows the decision tree and the likelihood of each outcome. The desired outcome is a successful operation with total relief of pain. In this case the highest possible number of QALYs is the same as the life expectancy for someone of his age, i.e. 15 years.

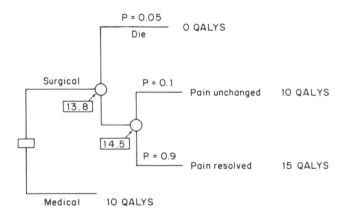

Figure 6.4   *Use of QALYs in decision analysis.*

To calculate the number of QALYs for a lifetime of persistent symptoms, the patient has to answer the question, 'What is the lowest number of years in perfect health that you would accept in exchange for your life expectancy with these persistent symptoms?' The patient may decide that 10 years of life with normal health would be equivalent to 15 years of life with persistent symptoms. The outcome with persistent symptoms is designated as 10 QALYs and the patient has made what is called a time trade-off, the decision having been made by the patient and not the doctor.

The decision tree can now be folded back in exactly the same way described in the previous example using QALYs instead of years. The average number of QALYs in those who have had the operation and survived is:

$$(0.1)(10) + (0.9)(15) = 14.5 \text{ QALYs}$$

This figure is then used to calculate the expected QALY at the next chance node. Clearly the best decision would be for claudication to be treated surgically in this particular patient.

There are more sophisticated ways of calculating QALYs than using the time trade-off method; for example, using the standard reference gamble which is described later. But, given the inherent weakness in using standard reference gambles, and the difficulty of explaining these to the patient, the time trade-off method is a more practical method.

In this particular example the QALY has been derived through a decision made by the patient, but in other cases the QALY is quantified from a combination of expected life span, from life tables, and a factor representing the survival quality. This ignores differences between patients in their approach to uncertainty and assessment of life values, and also evades the confounding factor of inter-individual variation. The average QALY may not apply to an individual patient who may be more physiologically sound than the average person of his age. A further, arguable, disadvantage is that the QALY concept gives preference to younger people with most years remaining, because the length of expected life is a major determinant. Some readers, particularly the younger ones, may feel this appropriate, but they may feel less comfortable about the inbuilt bias given to young, white, females from the upper social classes.

For this reason, and perhaps also because it belittles the wisdom of the doctor, the concept of QALYs has found more favour with health care planners than doctors, who remain sceptical. Quality of life is difficult and time-consuming to measure, but is it not reasonable to ask whether the alternative is better? When medical practice is based on accurate diagnosis and effective treatment, there are potential advantages to be gained in tailoring this to the individual patient. But when there is considerable uncertainty, the advantage may not be so obvious, and there can be no doubt that decisions may be based on illogical factors such as the doctor's own particular interest and the patient's ability to cause trouble.

COST EFFECTIVENESS ANALYSIS

However much we may dislike the idea of cost limiting the provision of health care, there can be no escaping the fact that there will never be enough money to provide perfect care for all. This puts the doctor in a difficult dilemma. On the one hand he is the patient's advocate in securing the best treatment possible irrespective of cost. On the other hand, he has the responsibility to make sure that the available finances are used to maximum benefit. Some doctors argue that accepting less than best for their patient is unethical, but this view is far too simplistic. It is equally unethical to deny another patient good care, but this happens when the use of resources is not adequately planned. Moving a patient out of a coronary care unit (CCU) to release a bed for a patient with a more pressing problem involves making a choice to optimize outcome with limited resources. The patient moved out of the CCU may still be at some risk, and have had a better chance of survival if close monitoring had been continued. The only way to avoid this would be to have enough CCU beds staffed to cover all eventualities. This could only be done by taking resources away from another department in which there may already be difficulties in providing adequate care.

Private health schemes are not exempt from financial pressure, although the physician's role of patient's advocate is more easy to fulfil in these circumstances. Eventually, soaring costs of health care will increase insurance premiums thereby pricing private health care out of the pocket of the less well off. Pre-paid health schemes—in which the physician is paid a lump sum to care for all of the patient's health needs—provides a strong incentive to avoid unnecessary expense, but the doctor's role as patient's advocate may conflict with self-interest when the practice budget, out of which his salary must come, is fixed.

These difficult dilemmas are not easy to solve, but should not be ignored. As health care costs soar there will be increasing pressure to take financial considerations into account and to use the most cost effective treatment. The term 'cost effectiveness', now in general usage, is derived from a branch of decision analysis which has been used in business for many years. Before looking at a simple example of such an analysis applied to medical practice, we should try to define what is meant by cost effectiveness, because the term is often used inappropriately or with an imprecision which makes it meaningless.

Sometimes the term refers simply to the cheapest or more effective treatment, and often the term is used vaguely when neither the cost nor effectiveness has been clearly defined.[75] In the health care field, the most cost effective treatment can be defined as the cheapest treatment for an equal or better health care outcome. This may be difficult to determine, but the situation may be complicated further by the availability of treatment which gives a worse outcome but is far cheaper. A definition purely in terms of cost per unit outcome is more all-embracing, for example pounds per year of life, but this can be over-simplistic. To take an example: if treatment A costs £1000 and produces a life expectancy of five years, and treatment B costs £100 to produce a life expectancy of one year, the most cost effective approach would be to choose B which gives one year of life for £100 compared with A which gives one year of life for £200. Nevertheless, many people would still regard option A as a preferable outcome because the marginal cost effectiveness is also attractive. The marginal cost effectiveness is defined as:

$$\frac{\text{cost of A} - \text{cost of B}}{\text{LE of A} - \text{LE of B}}$$

which in this case would be £225 per year of life, a result which will be regarded as attractive in a financially well off country. The term cost effectiveness could be applied to this situation where the additional benefit can be regarded as worth the additional cost. Whether it is really worth the additional cost or not depends upon the wealth of the health care setting and the relative cost of treatments given for other conditions.

To take a further example; consider the cost and effectiveness of surgery compared with lithotripsy in the treatment of renal stones. The decision tree is shown in Figure 6.5 with possible outcomes for a relatively high risk case. When lithotripsy fails, the patient proceeds to surgery with possible cure or peri-operative death. Notice that there are now two different types

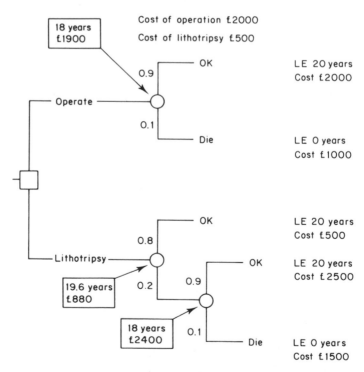

Figure 6.5   *Cost effectiveness of surgery compared with lithotripsy for renal stones.*

of outcome, one in terms of life expectancy and the other in terms of financial cost. It is possible to fold back the decision tree, as previously described, for cost and life expectancy separately. In this example, lithotripsy is a clear winner producing a longer life expectancy at a lower cost. If surgery had given a better survival figure, but at a higher cost, it would have been worth working out the marginal cost effectiveness to decide if the extra cost was worthwhile.

Life expectancy need not be one of the outcomes; it could equally well be QALYs, in which case the technique is known as cost utility analysis. The principles remain the same. Cost benefit analysis is sometimes confused with cost effectiveness analysis, but there is a crucial difference. Cost benefit analysis applies to the situation where both the cost and benefit are in the same terms, and these are usually financial. This means putting a monetary value on human life, which may include calculating the effect of a policy on the patient's lifetime earnings, or even on his use to society. The cost should also take into account such factors as the interest lost on the money spent on a treatment, and also the cost of any second treatment which may be necessary because the first was successful.[76] Because of difficulties inherent in doing this, cost benefit analysis has found only a limited role in health care.

Whilst most doctors do not readily accept this financial approach to medicine, the increasing difficulty in financing health care, which is not limited to poorer countries, may force it upon us. It is far better to take a realistic and honest view of the cost and benefit of medical care, than to practise medicine without regard to resources and with little evidence about outcomes. In the course of time, the economic approach may be seen as more effective, equitable and ethical.

ANALYSIS BY UTILITY

We have already seen an example of how a patient could participate in decisions about his own health when QALYs were described. The branch of decision analysis dealing with this is called 'utility analysis', utility being a quantitative measure of the strength of a patient's preference for an outcome. Utility analysis is a way of comparing gambles so that the gamble with the highest expected utility can be chosen by the patient. The method for comparing gambles was described by Oskar Morgenstern, an economist, and John von Neumann, a mathematician, and is based on what has been called the standard reference gamble. The technique of utility analysis is understood best by working through an example.

In this example, the problem faced is whether the patient's back pain, which is due to a prolapsed disc, should be treated by surgery or injection of the disc with papain. The troublesome symptom is that of persistent back pain, but there are no neurological sequelae. The decision tree is shown in Figure 6.6.

If surgery is undertaken the perioperative mortality is 5% (unrealistically high to make the figures simple). There are three possible outcomes in the patient who survives the operation: 80% are completely cured of the problem, but in 10% the problem persists, and in a further 10% the operation has been complicated

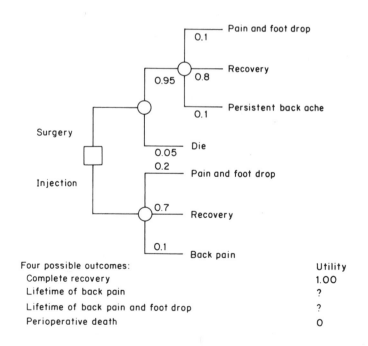

Figure 6.6 Decision tree comparing surgery with injection of papain for treatment of vertebral disc problems.

by damage to nerve roots leading to permanent foot drop as well as persistent back pain. The possible outcomes with injection are similar, except that perioperative death does not occur, and the probability of each outcome differs from those after surgery.

Utility varies from zero to one, zero being the worst possible outcome and one the desired outcome. It is easy to ascribe the value zero to perioperative death and one to complete recovery, but what is the utility for a lifetime of back pain and a lifetime of back pain together with foot drop? In each case this is decided after application of the standard reference gamble.

In the basic standard reference gamble, the patient faces a choice between a sure outcome and a procedure which has two possible outcomes. The ranking of the 'sure' thing' must be intermediate between the two potential outcomes of the procedures. The scenarios have then to be put to the patient, which is the most difficult and important aspect of utility analysis. The patient has to understand the options facing her and has to imagine situations which are both better and worse than her current predicament. In this case she is told that a sure thing is that without some form of treatment she is going to have persistent back pain for the rest of her life. An operation may cure the pain, but there is a significant risk of death. What chances of operative death would she take to be free of her pain?

This may be approached best by starting with a high probability of success and asking her if she would be prepared to take the risk. The answer would probably be yes. Then a low probability of success is chosen and the answer will probably be no. By adjusting the probability of success, eventually a probability will be chosen at which the patient is indifferent between the alternatives, the so-called 'indifference probability'. In this particular case the patient accepts a 5% risk of perioperative death. The utility is then calculated as shown in Figure 6.7.

The next standard reference gamble is a little more difficult for the patient to appreciate. She has to imagine that she has back pain and foot drop, but an operation could cure this, or, possibly, could prove fatal. In this case she should be prepared to take a higher risk and might settle for a perioperative death rate of 15% as the indifference probability. The utility for this then works out at 0.85.

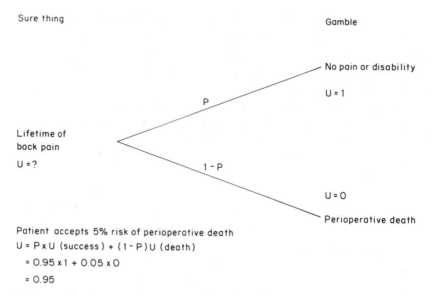

Patient accepts 5% risk of perioperative death
U = P x U (success) + (1 - P) U (death)
  = 0.95 x 1 + 0.05 x 0
  = 0.95

Figure 6.7 *Standard reference gamble for lifetime of back pain compared with surgical risks acceptable.*

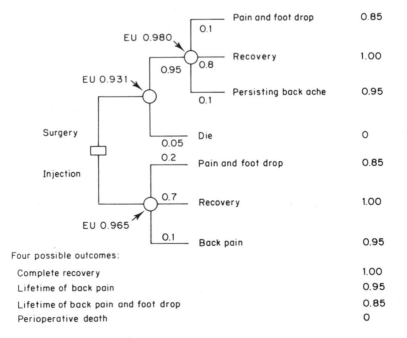

Figure 6.8 *Utility analysis comparing surgery with injection of papain for treatment of vertebral disc problems.*

It is now possible to put these utility figures into the decision tree (Figure 6.8) which can then be folded back as previously described. The expected utility (EU) at branch points is shown, and injection of the disc is the preferred option chosen by that patient. Another patient may prefer to take a higher risk of death rather than risk a failed procedure, in which case surgery may have the larger expected utility. Try the effect of putting in lower values of utility for pain and foot drop and persistent back pain.

Utility analysis can be used in more sophisticated ways than in this simple example. In many cases not only is the outcome state affected by the decision, but also the length of life. The patient may then have to make a decision about the risks she is prepared to take to achieve a certain state of health for a set time. These two aspects can be combined into a single utility for insertion into the decision tree. (The reader who has had a surfeit of decision analysis could skip this without losing the general gist of the chapter.)

An analysis of this sort is performed in two parts. First, the patient's attitude to length of life, and the risk he is prepared to take to maximize this, must be assessed. Secondly, a measure of the equivalence between length of life in ill health and length of life in normal health must be made.

To answer the first question, the doctor has to find out how willing a patient is to accept a quick death in the hope of achieving a normal life span. Consider the three situations shown in Figure 6.9. Twenty-five years is the expected normal life span of the patient, and this has the maximum utility of one. Immediate death has the lowest utility of zero. Suppose the patient is told that he has a 50% chance of achieving a normal life span and a 50% chance of immediate death, but he can forfeit the gamble and accept a minimum number of years which are guaranteed. If he is a logical person he should accept 12.5 years because this is the average life expectancy given a 50% gamble between 25 years and immediate death. Most people prefer not to take risks so he might accept a minimum 7 years of definite healthy life as equivalent to a gamble (Figure 6.9B) which might result in him dying immediately. Another person would accept a different figure.

He is now asked to consider the situation whereby he has a 75% chance of achieving a normal life span compared with a 25%

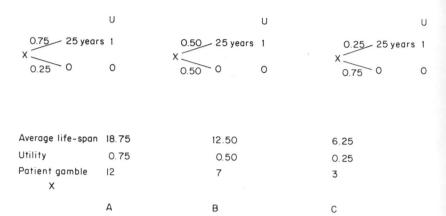

Figure 6.9   *Calculation of a patient's attitude to risk taking. X = the minimum number of guaranteed years that patients will accept to avoid the gamble between immediate death and a full life at different levels of risk 0.25, 0.50, 0.75.*

risk of immediate death when the average life expectancy would be 18.75 years (Figure 6.9A). Clearly, he would want a higher guaranteed figure than 7 years; in this case 12 years. In Figure 6.9C the odds are changed, and the average life expectancy is 6.25 years, but the patient, who is averse to risk, accepts the guaranteed 3 years.

It is now possible to draw a utility curve with the utility, calculated as shown in Figure 6.9, plotted against the years of guaranteed healthy life the patient considers equivalent (Figure 6.10A). The solid line shows the curve of this patient who tends to avert risk. The dotted line shows the curve of a patient who is neither averse to risk nor seeks it—the logical person— and the dashed line shows the curve of a relatively rare patient who seeks risk in the hope of achieving a full life span.

The next step is to measure the equivalence between length of life in a certain state of ill health, and length of life in normal health. This could be made using the simple trade off method previously described, or by using a standard reference gamble. A possible result is shown in Figure 6.10B along with the utility curve for the patient (Figure 6.10A). The purpose of the exercise is to derive a utility figure, combining length of life and state of health, so that it can be incorporated into the decision tree.

It may, for example, be a number of years with persistent back pain and foot drop in the example previously discussed. The

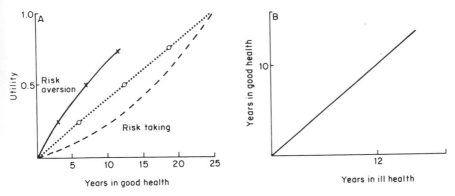

Figure 6.10 *A: Relationship between utility and years in good health calculated as described in the text and shown in Figure 6.9. The solid line is derived from the figures calculated in Figure 6.9 and represents a patient who is adverse to risk. The dotted line shows the relationship in a perfectly logical patient and the dashed line the relationship in a person who positively seeks risk in the hope of achieving a cure. B: trade off which a patient might make between years in ill health as against a lower number of years in perfect health.*

question may be, 'What utility value should be assigned to a life of 12 years with these symptoms?' From Figure 6.10B the number of equivalent years in good health is found first and the value of 10 years is obtained. This value is then put into Figure 6.10A to give the final combined utility value. For a patient who averts risk in the way defined by the utility curve shown, the utility value for 12 years of persistent back pain and foot drop would be approximately 0.7. This value can then be inserted into the appropriate branch of the decision tree and the whole process repeated for the different outcome state of persistent back pain without foot drop. The utility curve would be the same, but the equivalence between years in good and ill health (Figure 6.10B) would be different. This value can then be inserted into the appropriate part of the decision tree and the analysis completed.

The purpose of these examples is to give an impression of the potential power of utility analysis. It is possible to take it further, for example, to combine the concept of utility analysis and Bayes' theorem to evaluate whether a test should be performed. This involves not only whether the result of the test is likely to alter management, but also whether the patient is prepared to take the risk of the investigation to achieve that. In some cases there may be two possible investigations, one less invasive but also less accurate, and the patient could choose what risk he is prepared to take to be more certain of the diagnosis. Such evaluations are relatively complex, but may be justified in special circumstances like neurosurgery, where the risks of some investigations and inappropriate treatment are both clear cut and high.

LIMITATIONS AND ATTRACTIONS OF DECISION ANALYSIS

Some of the problems discussed in relation to the use of Bayesian statistics also apply to decision analysis. In particular, the shortage of appropriate numerical information to fit into the decision tree and the time required to use the method are both serious drawbacks. As with Bayesian statistics, the concepts of decision analysis have been understood for many decades, but they have not found wide acceptance.

The attraction of the approach is that it provides a way of ensuring the best chance of a good outcome. What will happen to the individual patient cannot be predicted with certainty, but in the absence of an invariable causal connection between treatment and result, an optimal outcome is all that can be hoped for. Given the uncertain results of treatment and the risks involved, should the patient not have the major say in what line of management is to be adopted, as in utility analysis?

Although this is an attractive idea, it is one that is particularly open to question. There are no doubt some patients who like to be directly involved in these decisions, and this may be influenced by national temperament, but the majority of people have difficulty in remaining rational when their health is involved, particularly if the illness is serious and outcome dependent upon a risky gamble. A rational approach to decision making is often forsaken when personal gambling is involved.[77] For example, the way the options are presented (the framing) has a strong influence on the gamble taken. Patients look much more favourably on an operation which guarantees 90% survival rather than 10% mortality. A glass half full is preferred to a glass half empty. This irrational tendency is not limited to the patient who has most to lose by a wrong decision; physicians show a similar weakness[78-80] even when supplied with all the appropriate facts and probabilities.

In fact, most people do not wish to take risks, choosing options which appear not to be gambles at all. There is an illogical preference for a gamble about which there is definite information even when the alternative, on average, may be better. A 30% chance of cure is likely to be preferred to a 0–80% chance of cure. Most people are risk averters when it comes to health, even though they may be willing to take unnecessarily high risks when it comes to interests such as rock climbing and parachuting.

Given this tendency for man to be irrational, it could be argued that personal decision making should be avoided. This view is hard to defend, but if a patient does not wish to take the responsibility of a gamble on his own health, alternatives to utility analysis such as life expectancy analysis allow the optimum outcome to be predicted. If it can be shown by sensitivity analysis that patient preference does not materially influence the outcome over a wide range of values, there is less reason to involve the anxious patient in these difficult decisions. But, at the very least, a doctor should seek a decision which follows these rational lines rather than impose his own views of risk taking on the patient.

Whatever difficulties there are in the widespread use of decision analysis,[81] the emphasis it puts on decision making as a gamble is an important lesson for young doctors in particular. Rather than trying to seek diagnostic certainty in vain by asking for more and more tests, doctors should learn to accept that a confident diagnosis may not be possible. Indeed, it may not make any material difference whichever management choice is made—the choice may simply be a 'toss up'.[82]

One potential weakness of a decision analysis approach is the reduction of the clinical problem to a relatively simple decision tree. Whilst it is possible, in principle, to draw up a decision tree to suit an individual patient's problem, it is far more convenient and practical to use decision trees which are applicable to groups of patients. The simplification which this entails can introduce errors. However, the alternative may be no more accurate unless reliable facts, applicable to an individual patient's illness, are available. The disadvantage of simplification may be more apparent than real, and the advantage of a simple decision tree is that it makes the collection of appropriate and accurate information for future use more practical.

Another criticism of formal decision analysis centres on what is regarded as the dehumanizing aspect of rational analysis. The quantitative character of this approach is somehow seen to conflict with the caring role of physicians. This is not an argument with which I can find much sympathy. Surely it is better to attempt an improvement in care by accepting uncertainty and optimizing decisions by statistical means rather than holding unrealistic hopes about the ability of doctors' decision making skills to influence an outcome beneficially. Utility analysis in particular, although not easy to implement, gives the opportunity for patients to be closely involved in decisions regarding their care. It is not suggested that they should be imposed on the unwilling patient, but it is an avenue of approach available for those who wish to take that path, and by no stretch of the imagination could it be regarded as dehumanizing.

No doubt one of the reasons why these techniques have not caught on more readily is the natural resistance to change. Doctors are no more prone to this weakness than anyone else, rather the converse, but there is undoubtedly some resistance to the introduction of new ideas which are alien to the ethos instilled in the medical profession. The fact that these methods are numerical rather than explanatory adds to the difficulties— patients do not always accept decisions based on statistical facts, preferring a mechanistic explanation for the decision, however spurious that explanation may be.

Despite the difficulties and weaknesses involved in applying these rational methods to medical care, there are several real and potential advantages to them. Above all they demand a reasoned and systematic approach to medical problems with the formulation of precise questions. If the probabilities are not available to fulfil the requirement of the method, at least these techniques point to which questions should be asked. There is really no short cut if the precision of medical decision making is to be improved. Potentially, these approaches lead to efficient use of resources aiming at the optimization of outcome whilst providing quality and consistency of care. These cannot be bad goals. Those who dismiss these methods as irrelevant to medical problems should ask themselves how else uncertainty can be reduced.

The potential advantage of decision analysis was demonstrated in a study in which six surgical problems were reviewed by a group of fifty surgeons.[83] Their views were sought as to the best approach to the problem using conventional clinical reasoning, and this was compared with the best option derived from decision analysis, both using the best estimate of probability from the literature and those provided by the experience of the surgeon.

If it is agreed that the analytical assessment based on the best available estimates of probability was the correct one, it was shown that the surgeons' traditional approach was far from optimal. In only 59% of cases did the conventionally derived opinions of the surgeons coincide with the decision arrived by analysis. The major source of error was the inaccuracy of subjective estimates of probability, but inaccurate reasoning was also partly to blame.

Anyone who has practised medicine with an open mind must have felt uncomfortable about some of the diagnoses and management decisions made. This analytical approach to decision making does not remove the random element in health care outcomes, but it is a rational approach to optimizing decisions. As such it should alleviate the discomfort of decision making and be accepted as an important branch of medical science.

FURTHER READING

Bursztajn, H. J., Feinbloom, R. I., Hamm, R. M. and Brodsky, A. *Medical Choices; Medical Chances*. New York: Routledge, 1990.

Drummond, M. F. *Providing Health Care*. Oxford: Oxford University Press, 1991.

Knoebel, S. B. *Perspectives in Clinical Decision Making*. New York: Futura Publishing Company, 1986.

Seedhouse, D. *Liberating Medicine*. Chichester: John Wiley & Sons, 1991.

Sox Jr, H. C., Blatt, M. A., Higgins, M. C. and Marton, K. I. *Medical Decision Making*. Stoneham: Butterworths, 1988.

7
Limitations of Statistics

'Hardly anything is said by one writer the contrary of which is not asserted by some other.'

Descartes

INTRODUCTION

It soon becomes apparent to any doctor that ideas on the management of disease change at a rate which is both alarming and bewildering. This could be looked upon as a welcome sign of healthy progress, yet many an acclaimed breakthrough has been unsubstantiated by further studies, and what was deemed mandatory a few years ago may now be contra-indicated. Although the swings of opinion are not always so extreme, doctors who have been practising for any length of time are left feeling like observers standing on the seashore watching the tide of opinion coming in and out, whereas younger doctors, who have not yet experienced these swings of opinion, are in the happy position of remaining confident in their knowledge. Why is it that medical research often leads to disputed opinion rather than incontestable facts?

One of the major problems is the difficulty encountered in dealing with complex biological organisms, particularly if there is the extra ethical dimension of experimentation on humans. Ideally a research worker should be able to study the effect of changing just one variable, keeping other influences on the outcome constant. This is rarely possible, so to cope with this difficulty Fisher developed two related but different concepts, namely the controlled and randomized experiment. Both these are designed to neutralize the effect of variables not under study. In a controlled experiment the factors known to influence the outcome are purposely distributed equally in the two groups. Not that this is always easy to achieve and, moreover, the assumption has to be made that all important influencing factors are known. In a randomized experiment, on the other hand, the experiment is so arranged that the numerous influences on the outcome should cancel each other out, save for the variable under consideration.

Epidemiological studies are particularly difficult to undertake without there being some unwanted difference between the groups under study. Differences between the groups may not matter if they are likely to be irrelevant to the question under investigation. It is the so-called confounding variables which are far more important. For example, in the evaluation of a possible relationship between taking the contraceptive pill and the rate of cervical carcinoma, it would be important to know the number of sexual partners of those women included in the trial: since this could influence the incidence of cervical carcinoma, it is clearly a confounding variable. If a relationship between taking the contraceptive pill and cervical carcinoma was found it might be due to women on the contraceptive pill having more sexual partners—the real association could be with the number of sexual partners rather than with the contraceptive pill.

On the other hand, although religion might influence the decision about taking the contraceptive pill, it is unlikely to be a causative factor in cervical carcinoma. Therefore, religion is not a confounding variable even though it might be related to the incidence of cervical carcinoma through its association with the likelihood of being on the contraceptive pill. If the two groups, one without cervical carcinoma and the other with, differed significantly in religious beliefs it would not matter, but if they differed in sexual habits this could be relevant to any differences in the incidence of cervical carcinoma found.

The concepts of the controlled and randomized trial have proved to be powerful tools in statistical analysis, but they are not without weaknesses. One unfortunate twist of fate is that on completion of a randomized study it may be apparent that an influencing factor has escaped randomization, and this could even escape attention if the influence is not recognized. Whilst it is reasonable to assume that the effectiveness of treatment is not going to be modified by the colour of the physician's socks, there can be important effects on the outcome which are not immediately obvious. For such reasons, Howson and Urbach[84] argue that the philosophical basis of randomization is not really sound, and that a surer basis is provided by Bayesian statistics. Be that as it may, the principle of randomization still dominates medical research.

One response to this problem of dealing with the complex interaction between man and disease is to choose to do laboratory research, often on animals, in order to achieve closer experimental control. Sometimes discoveries made with this approach are of profound importance to an understanding of the cause and expression of human illness, but often the findings are less relevant to the treatment of disease. When it comes to the management of disease in the ill patient, there is no escaping the need for large studies in which the confounding factors can somehow be eliminated. In most situations all one can hope for is a sound statistical statement relating a specific form of management to outcome. It may not be possible to say how a particular patient will respond to treatment, but it should be possible to give the average outcome if 100 patients were so treated. An accurate statistical approach is a perfectly sound basis on which to practise medicine in the absence of certainty. The problem is that the statistical base is often not sound, and most of this chapter will be directed towards examining why this may be so.

It was Disraeli who said that there are three types of lies: lies, damned lies and statistics. This dismissive view of statistics results not from a weakness in statistical theory, but from a lack of understanding as to what statistics have to offer and its consequent misuse, as demonstrated by the surgeon who told his patient not to worry about the mortality of the proposed operation being 50% because the last 50 patients all died. It is relatively easy to use statistical formulae—all one has to do is to look up the details in a book of statistical methods and put the data into a simple equation; nowadays, it is even simpler with the use of an appropriately programmed computer. However, the crucial part is in picking the test which is appropriate to the circumstances and which can answer the question asked. This means that a study should be designed with a view to limitations imposed by the statistics; most studies fall down in the design stage and these are irredeemable. This is most readily seen in the need to calculate the number of patients required to give a reasonable chance of finding a significant difference between one treatment and another.

Fortunately, the statistical design of studies has improved remarkably over the last twenty years; in part, this is due to the acceptance of statistical advice. No longer are parametric methods such as t tests applied when the data available is insufficient to guarantee a normal distribution, or when the data involves ordinal rather than interval scales. In these circumstances, a non-parametric method such as a Wilcoxon or Mann–Whitney test is more appropriate, and most research workers are aware of this. If not, it is unlikely that their paper will pass the scrutiny of the referees. There is also a growing recognition of the importance of confidence intervals when expressing the results of comparative trials which allows a more realistic appraisal of the value of treatment than does the use of P values. Above all, there is an increased trend to involve professional statisticians in medical research, particularly with large clinical trials. Although in doing so there is always a danger in a statistician who knows nothing about medicine talking to a physician who knows nothing about statistics, this trend is to be welcomed.

There are many potential pitfalls for the research worker involved in clinical research and it is possible only to give an outline of such problems in this chapter. The first difficulty considered is one which is peculiar to human experimentation— the possible placebo effect of any form of treatment. To overcome this it is desirable to compare the response to any new treatment with the response to a placebo. But this can present problems of its own. For example, when there is an accepted treatment for a condition it may be considered unethical to use a placebo. In these circumstances it is more proper to compare the new treatment with the accepted approach. However, unless one type of treatment has been compared directly with a placebo at some time, there is always a danger of simply comparing one placebo effect with another, neither treatment having a physical effect.

As well as being important in the assessment of treatment, comparison of outcomes between groups may also be useful in investigating the cause of disease, particularly in an epidemiological setting. When two groups are similar save for one particular feature, for instance cigarette consumption, then any differences in outcome are likely to be due to this feature, directly or indirectly. This basic logical truth is stated in John Stuart Mill's canon of difference, previously mentioned in Chapter 2. But for whatever reason the comparison is made, it is obviously essential that the two groups are truly comparable; that is, they can be regarded as belonging to the same population, in the statistical sense, except for the specific feature under investigation. This need for truly comparable groups is one of the major problems in medical statistics because of the ease with which bias so easily creeps in. Nevertheless, whatever statistical limitations there may be, there can be no doubt that the large randomized prospective trial is deservedly popular. The size of such trials should ensure a very good chance of detecting a significant difference between groups if such a difference really exists. Also, a well planned trial of this type is likely to be published whatever results are obtained. However, there are limitations even to this approach, some of which have already been touched upon, and these will be explored further in this chapter.

Some problems are intrinsic to the statistical method. One of these is the possibility of false positive results, the so-called type 1 error, which can occur however well a study is planned, performed and reviewed. Usually the chance of such an error is small, but publication bias can magnify this error to serious proportions. In contrast to this, false negative results—type 2 errors—in which a study fails to show a difference which really exists, may arise because there are too few subjects in each group. Given the difficulties in organizing large trials, it is hardly surprising that this is a common problem. By combining the results of several small studies, using the technique of meta-analysis, it may be possible to salvage some useful information. The problems of type 1 and 2 errors, along with the advantages and limitations of meta-analyses will be discussed.

THE PLACEBO EFFECT

When the term placebo is used correctly it refers to the psychological effect that an inert substance may have on the wellbeing of a person. Placebo means, 'I will please', and there can be no doubt that positive action pleases people even when there is little problem in the first place. In *The Pickwick Papers*, Charles Dickens relates how much better Mr Pickwick felt on taking the waters of Bath: 'After every fresh quarter of a pint, Mr Pickwick declared in the most solemn and emphatic terms, that he felt a great deal better; whereat his friends were very much delighted, though they had not been previously aware that there was anything the matter with him.' This desire to take medicine is peculiarly human, an observation which led Osler to comment on it as a way of distinguishing man from other animals.

In a study using medical students,[85] blue or pink sugar pills were given with the information that one type was sedative and the other a stimulant. Approximately two-thirds of the students taking the blue pill (supposedly a sedative) reported drowsiness, and one-third of the students taking the pink pill felt less tired. In all, one-third reported significant side effects, other than sedation or stimulation. This non-specific effect of a drug has led to the cynical view that one should treat as many patients as possible with a new drug whilst it still has the power to heal.

Because of this placebo effect, clinical studies involving treatment should have a control group taking a matched placebo whenever feasible. This may not be possible for ethical reasons where the type of management studied is a surgical operation, but inevitably the confidence in the physical effect of the operation will be correspondingly diminished. Despite these ethical objections there have been examples of studies published in which a control—sham—operation has been performed. Ligation of the internal mammary artery was once advocated for the relief of angina and many patients seemed to benefit. It had a brief vogue until 1959 when Cobb and his colleagues[86] showed that five out of nine patients who had a sham operation improved which compared with five out of eight patients who had the artery ligated. Whilst one cannot imagine this being passed by an ethics committee nowadays, it is salutary to consider that results of this and another similar trial led to the operation being abandoned after a brief lifecycle of two years. This may have saved many operative deaths, an observation which raises interesting ethical questions.

Not that one should regard a placebo controlled trial as an absolute requirement before a new treatment is accepted. When the results of treatment are remarkably good, as with the beneficial effect of penicillin, a control group may not be essential; but, unfortunately, the positive physical benefit of treatment is often not so definite. Given that a non-specific benefit will accrue from the placebo effect, the physical result of active treatment may be dubious. It has been said, no doubt with tongue in cheek, that the best way to improve the results of any treatment is to leave out the controls. The doctors benefit, the patients benefit and only science suffers![87]

When the effectiveness of a new treatment is not verified properly, there is always the danger of it becoming established in general usage inappropriately. This could explain why estimates show that over one-third of modern prescriptions are unlikely to have a specific pharmacological effect. Doctors as well as patients can be duped into thinking that a useless treatment is effective and, paradoxically, this may be advantageous. For whilst the placebo effect is the enemy of rational assessment, there can be no doubt that it is a powerful therapeutic weapon, but if the doctor does not believe in it some of the effectiveness is lost.

The positive benefit resulting from placebo treatment can raise difficult ethical problems. If the treatment is safe and inexpensive it could be regarded as unethical to deny the patient the benefit of it. The use of a sugar pill or an inert injection has its attractions, but even in the 19th century a doctor was successfully sued for injecting a lady with water instead of morphine, on this occasion on the grounds that she was charged for morphine. These days, our placebos are more expensive, partly because of the need to convince the doctor that something potentially effective is being given. Few areas in medicine are incontestable, but many treatments have dubious benefit. The occasional use of oxygen in patients with chronic airways disease is one example of an expensive treatment which may well have no physical effect. In some cases the placebo treatment may not even be safe. Despite this, there are few, if any, doctors who do not prescribe treatments in the hope for a response which could be only a placebo effect.

In evaluating treatment, the use of a control group is important not only because of the possible placebo effect of treatment, but also because disease can improve with the passage of time quite independently of therapy. There are, therefore, strong arguments in favour of a placebo group when treatment is being evaluated, and there are good reasons for both the patient and doctor being unaware of which treatment is given, as in the double-blind placebo-controlled trial. Clearly the patient should not know which treatment he is on, otherwise the effectiveness of the placebo would be negated. It is also desirable for the doctor to be unaware of which treatment is given if this is at all feasible, because he may indicate his own expectations to the patient quite unconsciously by his actions or approach.

RETROSPECTIVE VS. PROSPECTIVE STUDIES

Comparative studies are necessary not only for the evaluation of treatment, but also for estimating the usefulness of tests, and determining the cause of disease. The design of such studies varies considerably in detail, but they generally fall into two categories—retrospective and prospective. In both cases the quality of the trial depends upon the similarity of the groups compared. In an ideal study, they should be identical except for the feature under investigation, whether it be the effect of a drug or a possible cause of disease. The ideal situation is rarely if ever achieved in practice, but it is more nearly approached in randomized prospective trials. Some understanding of the differences between these approaches is therefore desirable.

Most doctors have some concept of what is meant by retrospective and prospective trials, and it is for this reason that I have retained the terms, even though they are not terms which currently find favour with epidemiologists. The alternative, and arguably better terms, of case control and cohort studies are less familiar but more accurate. These two contrasting methods for comparing groups can be understood in terms of the two rational approaches, the one inductive and the other hypothetico-deductive. The relationship between these terms is as follows:

retrospective = case = inductive = effect→cause
               control

prospective = cohort = hypothetico- = cause→effect
                                deductive

An example may help to clarify these contrasting approaches. In order to evaluate the benefit or otherwise of thrombolytic therapy in the treatment of acute myocardial infarction, the better approach would be to do a prospective study, randomizing all patients who have had a myocardial infarction into two groups, one being treated with thrombolytic therapy and the other not. In all other respects the groups should be similar, particularly in treatment used. In this case the hypothesis is made that thrombolytic therapy will reduce the mortality, and the purpose of the study is to put this hypothesis to the test. Each group is considered as a cohort which is followed in a positive direction in time. In that sense the study is prospective moving from presumed cause—thrombolysis of clots—to effect—reduced mortality.

The alternative retrospective approach would be to identify two groups containing patients who have had myocardial infarcts, one group comprising patients who died, and the other group patients who survived. The aim would then be to determine, by looking back in time, what differences in the two groups there might be to explain the different outcome. One of these variables could be the use of thrombolytic agents. If this therapy was used significantly more frequently in patients who survived, the inference might be that it was beneficial. However, such a retrospective study would be far from satisfactory. One of the many weaknesses could be that thrombolytic therapy was used more commonly in patients who were particularly ill, and this would strongly bias the results against showing any beneficial effect.

In other circumstances the case control or retrospective study would be more acceptable and sometimes more desirable because such studies are easier to mount. Often they can be concluded from what is simply good practice of routine data collection. One example of this approach would be a study looking into the cause of cervical carcinoma. Two groups could be evaluated, one group comprising patients who have cervical carcinoma and the control group who do not. Basic data on these patients should already be available so it is now possible to explore backwards in time—retrospectively—various differences in the two groups which might be relevant to the development of cervical carcinoma. The use of the contraceptive pill or the number of sexual partners are two of the possible causative factors which could be evaluated. This process of seeking from effect to cause is essentially an inductive process. To emphasize the opposing nature of the two approaches, Feinstein has called the case control method trohoc (cohort reversed).

The confusion in equating the terms retrospective and prospective with the case control and cohort approach arises because a cohort study can be performed on data which has been collected in the past, and, conversely, a case control study could be planned from data to be collected in the future. For example, to test the hypothesis that working with nickel increases the incidence of lung cancer, it would be possible to trace men working in certain factories using nickel many years ago, and then to compare the number developing lung cancer in this cohort with an equivalent cohort of workers who have not worked with nickel. Despite this being available from past data it is, nevertheless, a cohort study looking from possible cause to effect; in this sense it could be called a prospective study. Similarly, it would be quite possible and, in many cases desirable, to perform a case control study in the future by deciding to start collecting specific data on patients who have a particular disease, such as gall stones, with a view to comparing them later with a group who do not. This type of study would still be looking at the effect first with a view to determining the cause and in that sense would be retrospective.

When prospective is equated with a study moving forward, from cause to effect, and retrospective with a study moving backwards, from effect to cause, confusion need not arise. The terminology is important, because cohort studies are much less prone to bias than case control studies and, consequently, they are considered more scientifically respectable. The incorrect use of the term prospective may, therefore, give a study undue legitimacy and the smart research worker is aware that such studies are more popular with editors.

BIAS IN CLINICAL TRIALS

The problem of bias in the design and execution of clinical trials was considered in detail by Sackett[88]. He identified 35 biases which can arise, and looked at 9 of these in detail. Some of these biases apply to both retrospective and prospective studies, but all of them could influence the results of retrospective trials. They can be grouped into biases of sampling and measurement.

Sampling biases are particularly difficult to avoid. Patients included in a disease group may not, for example, be typical of patients with that disease. They are often chosen from patients admitted to hospital who will, therefore, tend to have the more severe features of the disease. Any conclusions drawn from such a study could only apply to this selected group, and this can make investigation of aetiological factors particularly difficult.

Another sampling problem is the selection which occurs when a significant proportion of subjects who have been sent questionnaires fail to reply. The responders and non-responders may differ in some important way which influenced their decision to respond. They may, for example, smoke and drink more heavily than the responders, and feel embarrassed about this, or resentful that the question has been asked. Any conclusions from such a questionnaire would then be heavily biased against the possible influence of these factors. It is difficult to achieve a 100% response rate, but every effort should be made to achieve at least an 80% response rate; otherwise the study may be meaningless.

An example of measurement bias is the effect of knowing a person's previous exposure to a suspected causative factor on the intensity of investigation for a particular disease. For example, routine tests in workers exposed to toxic chemicals could lead to a high diagnosis of cancer. Alternatively, when a patient is known to suffer from a disease, the search for the suspected causative factor may be more thorough. Questions about specific exposure to asbestos, for example, may be made more positively in people with pleural disease than in controls.

Although a prospective trial is likely to give an answer more reliably than does a retrospective trial, it is still necessary to avoid bias. It is essential, for exampe, to randomize the patients after inclusion in the trial, otherwise the physician may decide not to include the patient on one pretext or another. The reason for exclusion, perhaps unwittingly, could be an important influence on the outcome, and this influence would then not be distributed equally between the two groups. Alternatively, the patient's decision about giving consent may be influenced by the knowledge of the type of treatment to be offered. In both cases bias will be introduced.

Another way of avoiding bias is to analyse on an 'intention to treat' basis, to avoid bias introduced by taking patients out of the trial. For example, removal of patients from the treatment arm of the study because of complications caused by the treatment may result in the study showing a useful response to this treatment which is false. If the patients with complications had remained in the study, the overall effect of treatment may not have been beneficial. On an intention to treat basis, these patients would still be included in the treatment group. At the very least, the reasons for patients dropping out of the trial should be stated in the paper. If the reasons for dropping out do not seem relevant to the question asked of the study, the pragmatist would point out that they may be ignored. In that case fewer patients may need to be entered into the trial to show a positive effect.

It is worth saying that most of these biases should be obvious to anyone who takes the trouble to consider in more detail the methodology of a study—it is largely a question of common sense and an enquiring mind. Undoubtedly the methods section of a paper deserves greater attention than it usually gets.

LIMITATIONS OF PROSPECTIVE RANDOMIZED TRIALS

The positive features of prospective placebo-controlled randomized trials, particularly for the assessment of innovations in therapy, have already been discussed. They reduce, but do not eliminate, the possibility of bias in the interpretation of results, and overcome the placebo effect which can have such a powerful influence on the outcome of illness. But, despite the obvious attractions of this approach, and the many notable successes using it, there are problems both in the implementation and basis of such trials. The first problem is purely logistic. Anyone who has been involved in large controlled trials will have appreciated the difficulties in implementing the protocol. Patients and, for that matter, doctors, do not always do as they are told.

Sir Bradford Hill, who introduced and championed the medical use of the randomized controlled trial, related a conversation with a patient who had been included in such a trial: 'Doctor, why did you change my pills?' asked a randomized patient. 'What makes you think that I have?' was the reply. 'Well, last week when I threw them down the loo they floated, this week they sink!'

There is also the question of pure numbers; in this regard it is important to make a distinction between the trial of a remedial therapy and the evaluation of prophylaxis. All patients put into a trial of remedial therapy would have the indication for the treatment. On the other hand, with prophylactic treatment only a small number of patients included in the trial may be expected to develop a complication of disease. The numbers needed in a prophylactic trial are, therefore, correspondingly greater. For example, the number of patients required to show that an antihypertensive agent is effective in lowering the blood pressure—remedial therapy—is much smaller than the number required to show a definite fall in the incidence of myocardial infarction, stroke or renal failure which may result from a drop in the blood pressure—secondary prophylaxis.

The large number of patients required in the evaluation of prophylactic therapy usually makes it necessary to organize a multicentre trial with all the problems that entails. The coordination of such trials is a major commitment, and many trials may become impossible to complete because not enough patients, investigators or finance are available. Because the target to be prevented may not occur for many years after treatment is started, the problems are compounded by the need to keep the patient under observation for a protracted period. Over this time other promising treatments may become available and it may then be regarded as uninteresting, if not unethical, to continue with the study, so the question posed is never adequately answered. If subsequent developments prove less than satisfactory, an important opportunity may have been lost, or at least delayed, until a further study of the original treatment can be restarted and completed.

Despite these difficulties, and the problems of bias previously mentioned, it is possible, by means of the controlled randomized trial, to achieve a precise answer to a specific question posed with a high degree of certainty. However, to achieve this, the trial designers will have to be very fastidious in their approach. Paradoxically, this may lessen the usefulness of their results, and some argue that a pragmatic approach is more appropriate. If a trial is restricted to a tightly defined group, the results of the trial may only apply to those limited circumstances. The alternative pragmatic approach may lead to results in which less confidence can be held, but which may be more appropriate to the mixture of problems met in clinical practice. Accuracy is reduced for the sake of the results being more widely applicable.[89]

The more precise approach may be needed to answer specific questions about the causal connection between treatment and response. As an example of this, consider a trial in which the effectiveness of radiotherapy in combination with surgery is to be compared with surgery alone as a treatment of a particular cancer. To answer the question as to whether radiotherapy itself changes the outcome, it would be necessary to subject the non-radiotherapy group to a time delay between diagnosis and surgery equal to the time needed for radiotherapy in the treated group. Otherwise any improvement in outcome resulting from radiotherapy might be offset by the increased time delay between diagnosis and surgery, and the effect of radiotherapy would not be seen. What you gain on the swings, you stand to lose on the roundabouts.

A study designed in that way could give a precise answer as to whether radiotherapy has a positive effect on the tumour, but it would fail to answer the pragmatic clinical question as to whether radiotherapy should be given before surgery. In practice, radiotherapy will inevitably delay surgery, so the question the clinician wants answered is whether radiotherapy followed by surgery gives a different result from early surgery without radiotherapy. In this case, the time delay between surgery and radiotherapy would be incorrect, as well as being unethical.

The fastidious approach generates a further problem, namely the need for hard data such as death as the outcome end-point. In the evaluation of therapy for the secondary prevention of further cardiac events after a myocardial infarct, the cleanest outcome to look at would be further deaths due to infarction. But since these are relatively few a lot more data would be required than if the outcome was widened to include any ischaemic events, but a disadvantage is that these events will be more difficult to define precisely.

A further contrast in approach can be seen in the precision with which subgroups are analysed. The pragmatist may analyse patients with different degrees of compliance to medication, or with different control of end-points such as blood pressure, in separate groups, whilst the fastidious worker would lump these together to avoid bias. However, subgroup analysis not included in the design of the study is inherently weak—if enough subgroups are analysed some false difference is likely to be found because of random variability. On the other hand, in grouping the data together, the fastidious worker loses potential information, and the only way round this would be to mount studies with different levels of dosage and effect. This raises not only practical problems, but also ethical problems in that this approach would entail treating some patients with a dosage of a drug considered non-optimal, or titrating to an end-point which is thought less than ideal.

There is no universally right or wrong approach to randomized trials. For some questions a more fastidious approach is appropriate, but in other circumstances a pragmatic view should be taken. Some workers would rather accept more uncertainty for the sake of wider applicability. Others incline towards a more precise answer, but to a more limited question. In either case considerable investment is made when controlled trials are undertaken; it is, therefore, important that the question asked is relevant and likely to remain so for some time. In the long run, trials which lead to confidence in more general results may well prove more useful. Knowing that a specific anti-hypertensive agent at a specific dose reduces the risk of myocardial infarction is useful information, but knowing that several anti-hypertensive agents have the same effect would be even more relevant. It would be impractical to mount a precise trial for every type of anti-hypertensive agent or to check that every minor change in a therapeutic agent leaves the effectiveness unaltered.

By and large I have avoided ethical issues in this book, but mention should be made of an ethical dilemma presented by randomized trials. This arises from the conflicting demands of a moral theory based on the rights of an individual, such as expounded by Kant, compared with the utilitarian approach of

John Stuart Mill. It is valid to argue that when the best approach to a problem is questionable it is acceptable and even desirable to compare two treatments or, alternatively, one dubious treatment with a placebo. The information given by the study can be used for the greater good of future patients. However, an individual patient in the trial may be put at a disadvantage. There is the inconvenience of the trial with the extra attention and investigations which the study may well entail. Perhaps more importantly, there could be loss of confidence in the doctor. It is hardly encouraging when a doctor admits that he does not know how best to treat your illness and, moreover, the possible benefit of the placebo effect is lost. Discussing randomization can leave a patient bewildered and frightened.

As with most ethical issues there is no easy solution to this dilemma, but it has to be accepted that much of the current uncertainty in medical practice arises because the best approach has never been determined by a proper scientific trial in the first place. Even the benefit of anticoagulants in thromboembolic disease has not been proven in a rigorous sense, but there are few if any physicians who would not use them. There are many practices of more doubtful use which are nevertheless generally accepted. Once a practice is established it becomes virtually impossible, on ethical and legal grounds, to go back and rigorously test it. Obviously, it is highly desirable to determine the truth in the first place rather than to let dubious practices become established facts. It is hard enough to pinpoint the truth without succumbing to this ethical straightjacket.

TYPE 1 ERROR—FALSE POSITIVE RESULTS

When two groups are compared with a view to detecting a significant difference between them, as they would be, for example, when an active treatment is compared with a placebo, the null hypothesis is tested. In doing this the assumption is made that the two groups may contain figures from the same distribution even though the means appear to differ. If this difference results purely from random variability, the null hypothesis will be confirmed. Alternatively, the difference may be due, at least in part, to the effectiveness of the treatment, in which case the difference is likely to be so large that the null hypothesis is no longer tenable, and the effectiveness of the treatment will have been demonstrated. However, it is impossible to establish this with absolute confidence, and the limit of this confidence is stated by the P value. If the P value is 0.01 there is only a 1% likelihood that the difference is due to chance variation which means that, on average, in 100 studies demonstrating a significant difference at this level, there will be one publication which gives a false positive result.

If this were the sole problem, most people would regard it as irritating, but manageable. However, the problem is seriously compounded by our preference for positive results. In response to this, there is a strong bias towards publishing positive findings, first looked at objectively by Sterling[90] in a review of articles published in the *Journal of Experimental Psychology* in 1959. In those articles in which significance testing had been used, 105 out of 106 papers showed significant results at the 5% level. It has subsequently been shown that both the decision to submit articles for publication, and the decision to publish them, are strongly in favour of articles with positive results.[91] In one review, 82% of articles with a positive outcome were submitted compared with 43% with negative outcomes: out of these, 80% of the positive articles were accepted, but only 50% of the negative ones.[92]

Quite apart from the editorial response to public demand, there are several other reasons why the literature contains an unusually large proportion of papers with positive results, and, since this effect on our store of knowledge is so profound, it is worth enumerating them.

Retrospective vs. Prospective Studies

Published retrospective studies show a particularly strong bias towards papers with positive results. This was documented in a paper published by Sacks et al. (1983)[93] from which Figure 7.1 is taken. As an empirical finding this has to be accepted as strong evidence that this occurs, but one can only speculate as to why this might be so. A reason could be that the absence of blinding results in poor selection of controls; another might be selective withdrawal of study subjects, which is more difficult to do in a

Therapy	Randomized trials		Historical control trials	
	New treatment effective	New treatment ineffective	New treatment effective	New treatment ineffective
Coronary artery surgery	1	7	16	5
Anticoagulants for acute myocardial infarction	1	9	5	1
Surgery for oesophageal varices	0	8	4	1
Fluorouracil (5-FU) for colon cancer	0	5	2	0
BCG immunotherapy for melanoma	2	2	4	0
Diethylstilboestrol for habitual abortion	0	3	5	0

Figure 7.1 *The number of published clinical trials for six medical issues: comparison of randomised trials with trials using historical controls. From Sacks et al. (1983), with permission.*

randomized prospective double-blind study. Also, it is more difficult and time consuming to perform prospective trials, which adds to the determination to submit them for publication when the results are negative. Furthermore, editors are aware of the weaknesses inherent in retrospective studies and are even less inclined to publish a negative study with historical control.

Small Studies

Small studies are notoriously prone to show positive results and, again, publication selection is likely to be one of the main causes. In fact, small studies should be less likely to show a positive result because they have less potential power to do so. This point will be made again when looking at false negative results; the effect of this should be to produce a plethora of small studies with negative results, but the converse happens.

The funnel graph, in the hypothetical example shown in Figure 7.2, demonstrates this point visually. The graph of effect size against sample size should be symmetrical. The true difference between the groups, with an infinite sample size, is at the point of the funnel. The larger studies should be near the tip of the funnel. Smaller studies could be anywhere in the funnel with effect size evenly distributed around the true effect. When similar publications are plotted on this type of graph, there is

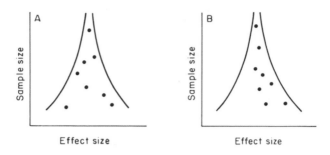

Figure 7.2   *Funnel graph comparing the effect sizes with sample sizes in a series of hypothetical publications concerning similar research, e.g. a drug effect. Publication bias leads to an asymmetrical distribution, as shown in B, with a tendency to publish results which show a large positive effect.*

usually a strong bias towards the more positive results giving graphs similar to Figure 7.2B.

Data Dredging

A further bias towards positive findings results from the statistical sin of data dredging. In the search for positive results authors may try different statistical tests or perform inappropriate subgroup analysis until a positive result is found. In prospective studies, the groups to be compared are decided in advance, and the whole design of the study is based on this. It is a fundamental error to seek subgroups which may, by chance, show a significant difference. These subgroups were not part of the null hypothesis in the first place. Statistical tests provide a basis for probability statements only when the hypothesis is fully developed before the data is examined, otherwise the P values may be very deceptive.

Study Selection

Whilst many research workers are strongly motivated by a desire to push back the boundaries of knowledge, there are many others who seek publications as a means of furthering their career. Inevitably, therefore, they will wish to do research which is likely to have a positive result and be publishable. Unfortunately, this attitude discourages potentially more important research work which may have a low chance of success or just show negative results.

Financial Incentives

Even more alarmingly there is the possibility that financial incentives may play a role in determining whether studies are undertaken and published. Given human nature this type of bias would not be surprising, and there is evidence that this does occur. In a review of clinical trials published in medical journals in 1984, 89% of trials which were supported by the pharmaceutical industry had positive results in favour of the new treatment, whereas only 61% of trials not so supported showed positive results.[94] Also, the proportion of controlled trials showing evidence of adverse drug effects is considerably higher in unpublished reports than amongst published work.

The strong bias towards positive results leads to an attitude of cynicism and incredulity towards drug trials, particularly those promoted by drug companies. It will be pointed out by those promoting a new drug that the P value is less than 0.01 and, therefore, the new treatment must be more effective than the old treatment with which it has been compared. If you complain about the sample size being small, you will be told that the statistics correct this. Don't believe a word of it: the bias introduced by small studies discussed here cannot be corrected by statistical manipulation—bias should be avoided in the first place by performing properly controlled clinical trials including an adequate number of patients. Even this will not guarantee a lack of bias, and it has been suggested that there should be a register of all planned trials so that unpublished trials can be available. It would also be helpful if editors published only those studies which are adequately designed; perhaps papers should be reviewed purely on the basis of the method.

TYPE 2 ERROR—FALSE NEGATIVE RESULTS

This type of error arises when the number of patients entered into a trial is insufficient to demonstrate a difference between the two groups even when a real difference does exist. Given random variability it is likely that there will be overlap in outcome between, say, treatment and non-treatment groups. The number of patients required to show a true difference between the two groups depends upon:

1. The degree of variability in the data.
2. The minimum size of the difference in the relevant measurement, for example blood pressure, which is regarded as being clinically useful.
3. The significance level sought (usually 1% or 5%).
4. The power of the study, i.e. the chance of obtaining a significant result if the two groups are truly different at the minimum specified level. Powers of 80% or 90% are typical choices.

When these are known or assumed, it is possible to calculate the number of patients required to demonstrate the difference sought if it really exists. If the difference is not found when the results are analysed, you can be reasonably confident that there is no true difference between the groups. However, if the study is performed with fewer than the required number of patients, it may well give a negative result, even when the two groups really differ. The study never had the power in the first place to answer the question posed.

Whilst many studies have been embarked upon which never had the potential power of giving a clear answer, it is true to say that there will be a strong bias against publishing these. Negative studies involving small numbers of patients are, quite understandably, not popular with editors, so type 2 errors are less influential than type 1. They do, nevertheless, occur and should always be considered when two treatments are said to have similar effects. The problem is far from negligible, as shown in a review of 15 randomized double-blind trials concerning acute severe asthma, in which 12 had less than a 60% chance of detecting a true 25% difference between treatments.[95]

It is sometimes said that if a study fails to show a significant difference between groups at least the difference cannot be all that large or important. Whilst there is a grain of truth in this, it can be misleading. If the variability of the outcome measured is large, or if the event of interest, for example death in myo-cardial infarction, is relatively infrequent, then large studies may be needed to show what could be quite an important difference between two treatments.

Conversely, an adequate study may show a clear statistically significant difference between two groups which is, in practice, of little importance. In a large study carried out by the World Health Organization an increased risk of cervical cancer was shown in patients taking the birth pill.[96] The relative risk was 1.5, but when this is analysed in terms of life expectancy, the average reduction in life expectancy for women aged 20 to 24 was 11 days and only 7 days for women aged 30 to 34. The risk of passive smoking, when examined in this way, is also relatively small.

META-ANALYSIS

Over the last ten years increasing use has been made of a statistical technique in which data is combined from independent studies to obtain a better estimate of the overall effect of a particular procedure. Glass (1976) was the first to coin the term 'meta-analysis' to describe this,[97] but there had been a few publications before that date in which the technique had been used. The purpose is to make use of the information available in small trials by pooling data from several publications which have been designed to answer the same basic question. Reasons for wishing to do this would include:

1. To reduce the problem of type 2 error by increasing the number of patients involved and, thereby, the statistical power.
2. To improve estimates of effect size since the overall confidence interval would be reduced by increasing the data; i.e. a large study will give a better estimate of the true difference between the two groups.
3. To put the results of any one trial in perspective, so reducing uncertainty when reports disagree.
4. To allow more realistic subgroup analysis.
5. To reduce referral bias in the hope that the results will apply to a more representative cross section of patients.

The success of the meta-analysis depends very much on the choice of trials which are included. Needless to say, a thorough search of the literature is necessary and information about unpublished trials should be sought and considered for inclusion. Many people believe that only randomized controlled trials should be considered, and undoubtedly it is the method section—not the results—which should take prime consideration. Criteria have to be established to decide which studies are similar enough to be pooled; too much heterogeneity between trials will invalidate the statistical methods for data pooling. The range of patient characteristics, the treatment used, the means of diagnosis and the measurement of outcome must all be considered.[98,99] The reason for rejecting data should also be stated.

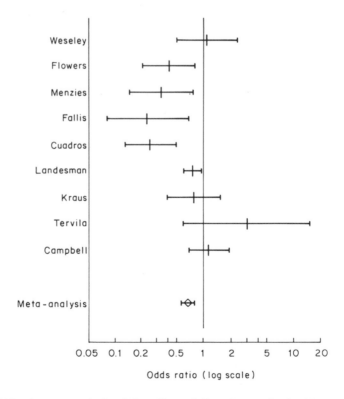

Figure 7.3   *A meta-analysis of the effect of diuretics on the incidence of pre-eclampsia. Odds ratios for pre-eclampsia and 95% confidence intervals in nine trials of diuretics. From the original data of Collins et al. (1985)[100] modified by Thompson and Pocock (1991) by permission of The Lancet Ltd.[102]*

There are many techniques for combining data from several trials which differ in detail. A common presentation is shown in Figure 7.3 which contains data from an overview of randomized trials examining the effectiveness of diuretics in reducing pre-eclampsia.[100] For each study the proportion of women suffering pre-eclampsia is shown for the diuretic and control group and the odds ratio calculated. This is the ratio between the number of patients who have pre-eclampsia and the number who do not for the treatment group compared with the control group. Effective treatment produces an odds ratio of less than one. The results are usually plotted on a logarithmic scale to make the confidence intervals symmetrical. Larger studies generally have a smaller confidence interval so the visual display can be misleading because the least informative trials dominate the graph.

An overall odds ratio can now be calculated which gives different weights to the various trials according to the number of patients included. A significance test can then be performed to check if this ratio differs significantly from one. Of the many different methods available, some do not distinguish small studies with large effects from large studies with small effects, and some do not yield an estimate of the size of the effect. The Mantel–Haenszel method,[101] and modifications of it, are currently the most popular techniques; they have the advantage of comparing each treatment group with its control, and they weight studies according to their size. For each trial the number of events in the treatment group is compared with the number expected if the treatment had no effect. The observed minus expected number are then totalled and a chi-squared test applied to check significance.

An assumption is made that the true treatment effect in each trial is the same. This may not be true particularly if, as is likely, the population and details of treatment differ. A formal test of statistical heterogeneity can be applied to test whether the treatment effects are more variable than can be ascribed to chance. If this is positive, and in the face of a meta-analysis which shows a significant effect of treatment, one is left with the difficulty in deciding to which trial circumstance or to which exact treatment this effect applies. It would be an unacceptable leap of faith to believe that the treatment is effective in all circumstances.[102]

Despite its advantages meta-analysis is not a substitute for a well planned and executed randomized prospective trial. None of the weaknesses resulting from publication bias are eliminated or even reduced by meta-analysis, unless it is possible to include data which has not been published. One question that may reasonably be asked is whether meta-analysis gives more precise information than a straightforward narrative review. Some critics are concerned that such an analysis could give an unwarranted sense of scientific validity simply because the comparative data is quantified. There is certainly some danger of that, but the demands of a systematic approach, and the quantitative comparison of data across the literature are in its favour. As with most things, the usefulness of a meta-analysis depends on how well it is done.

SUBJECTIVE PROBABILITY

The interpretation of medical data using statistical analysis is more subjective than might at first be appreciated. This was touched upon in Chapter 2 when it was pointed out that the type of statistics commonly used in medical research is based on frequential data such as the number of times a six is obtained when a die is cast one hundred times. On average, this will occur one out of every six throws, but this frequential data is only of limited use for the person who wishes to place a bet on the next throw. Next time it will either be a six or it will not, and if money is put on this, clearly it will be a gamble.

The same principle applies to the interpretation of findings from medical trials. You may be 95% certain that a trial shows streptokinase to be of use in acute myocardial infarction, but in making a decision to use streptokinase as a standard treatment in these circumstances, you are making a subjective decision. It is still quite possible, although less likely, that streptokinase is not effective, but a decision has to be made one way or the other and this is a subjective process.

This point may well be self-evident to the reader, but the implications are more subtle and deserve further consideration. One way of approaching this is to consider what is generally meant by the use of the word probable. When we say that it will probably rain tomorrow, we are saying that, from what we know about the current weather situation, and from our previous experience of it, we estimate that it is more likely to rain tomorrow than not. The probability of rain—P—is greater than 0.5; but this estimate at best can only be very approximate. It may, however, be the best we can do in the circumstances, and whether we cancel the trip to the seaside remains a subjective decision based on this.

Sometimes the probability may appear to be more precise. When it was said that there was a 95% chance of the first Apollo moonshot being successful, this information would have been based on considerable technical information giving it some respectability. However, it is not a really meaningful statistical statement except in the Bayesian sense of subjective probability. A true probability statement of $P = 0.95$ could only be made if there had been many identical moonshots before, and it had been found that 95% had arrived successfully. What is really being said is that the likelihood of the moonshot being successful is estimated to be the same as the likelihood of picking a white ball out of a bag containing 95 white balls and 5 red. A pseudo-frequential statement is being made.

The same is true when a trial is said to show that a new drug is significantly more effective than an old one. If the two treatment groups are significantly different at the $P = 0.05$ level, you could say that you were 95% certain that the new drug is more effective. However, this figure has been achieved by performing the experiment only once using two groups of patients. It has not been arrived at by performing the same experiment, say 100 times, to find that in 95 of these experiments a significant difference was found. All you can conclude is that your confidence in the new drug being more effective than the old drug is equal to your confidence in picking a white ball out of the same bag containing 95 white balls and 5 red ones, previously mentioned. Ultimately, the decision to use the drug or not is a subjective one.

Now, this might be thought to be somewhat academic; most people have a good feel for the likelihood of picking a white ball from the bag described. However, there is one very important implication and it is this: the probability of a hypothesis depends upon the prior probability of the hypothesis as well as the frequential probability of the observed data. The reasoning is similar, and some would say the same, as used in the application of Bayes' theorem to individual data. We can write Bayes' formula in the form

$$P(H|F) = \frac{P(F|H) \cdot P(H)}{P(F)}$$

where H stands for the hypothesis and F the experimental findings. This emphasizes the subjective nature of the final interpretation of the research work. It depends not only on the findings but also on the likelihood of the hypothesis in the first place, and this depends on prior knowledge.

To take a medical example for illustration: suppose a trial was performed which showed penicillin to be effective in the treatment of gout. This would seem highly unlikely from what we know about the pathogenesis of gout, so the prior probability of the hypothesis being true is very low; we might estimate this as 1%. Despite this, the study appears to show that penicllin is effective with the possibility of the null hypothesis being only 5%. From these results it would seem that we can be 95% confident that penicillin is an effective treatment of gout. However, this would still be very unlikely considering the low probability of this in the first place. The wise doctor would not rush into using penicillin for gout but would look at the study carefully or await further confirmation. In this case the accuracy of the diagnosis should be questioned; could a significant number of patients admitted into the trial have cellulitis and not gout would be one of the obvious questions to ask.

The Bayesian approach to statistics has been criticized because of the subjective nature of estimating the prior probability of disease. This is indeed a problem, but the influence of a mistaken estimate falls rapidly as the amount of data increases. Virtually all statistical methods used in medical research are based on Fisher's theory of significance testing and those of Neyman and Pearson. These were developed because of the subjective weaknesses inherent in Bayesian statistics, but subjective decisions have to be made when these theories are used. The conclusion of a study may differ according to which test statistic is used or, indeed, which null hypothesis is sought. The choice of probability level to which significance is attached, such as 0.05 or 0.01, is purely subjective. There is also the question of the choice of hypotheses which are to be considered admissible, and the influencing variables which are considered worth randomizing. As Howson and Urbach[84] point out, it is impossible to make statistics free of such subjective decisions.

A consequence of this subjective interpretation of experimental data is that even empirical science is never theory free. However hard we may try to put aside our hopes and prejudices we cannot, and perhaps should not, stop these influencing our beliefs. These subjective factors are implicit in our decisions about which hypothesis to accept and which to reject. The history of scientific discovery is entirely consistent with this; we work within paradigms, only abandoning an established theory when the weight of accumulated evidence against it is considerable.

FURTHER READING

Bradford Hill, A. *Principles of Medical Statistics*. London: The Lancet, 1966.

Feinstein, A. R. An additional basic science for clinical medicine. *Annals of Internal Medicine* 1983; **99**: 393–397, 544–550, 705–712, 843–848.

Gardner, M. J. and Altman, D. G. *Statistics with Confidence*. London: BMJ Publications, 1989.

Howson, C. and Urbach, P. *Scientific Reasoning: The Bayesian Approach*. La Salle, Illinois: Open Court Publishing, 1989.

Skrabanek, P. and McCormick, J. *Follies and Fallacies in Medicine*. Glasgow: The Tarragon Press, 1989.

Epilogue

The unifying theme running through the various topics of this book is the origin and management of uncertainty in medical practice. Students and young doctors often find uncertainty difficult to cope with particularly because of the heavy responsibility of dealing with people's lives, but eventually all must come to terms with it. Decisions have to be made; it is no good wearing oneself down trying to do the impossible and square the circle. It was Bertrand Russell who said, 'There is nothing more tiring than uncertainty, and nothing more futile.' Our aim must be to make the best decisions but on the understanding that, despite this, sometimes there will be undesirable outcomes. When the correct decision is unclear, it is as well to remember time honoured aphorisms such as 'First do no harm' and 'Common things occur commonly'.

In this book we have sought ways of reducing uncertainty, but no panacea has been discovered. The rewards resulting from the application of the scientific method to medical problems have been considerable, and there is no doubt that this approach will continue to lead to further understanding of disease with the attendant improvement in the treatment of patients. Basic research is essential, but there is an increasing need to apply our knowledge accurately to the ill person and, indeed, to the health of society as a whole. Our continuing uncertainty about the best management of common disease reflects badly on our approach. Too many studies are undertaken which do not address a useful question or do not have the potential power to answer the question posed. This wastes scarce resources, clutters the literature and confuses the unwary mind. Over the last twenty years there has been an increasing trend towards large well planned and well conducted clinical trials. Whilst these trials are not without their difficulties, and some of these have been discussed in this book, they are to be welcomed. Undoubtedly they will continue to make important contributions to management of disease in the future.

The accurate collection of data from patients should not, and need not, be limited to data from patients included in clinical trials. There is much to be learned from individual patients, but it is essential to collect relevant information accurately. This is a time consuming and, therefore, costly business, but if medical audit is to succeed, resources will need to be made available for this. The observation that one half of the improvement obtained using a computer aided diagnostic system was due to better collection of data emphasizes the potential improvement that could be achieved by doing simple things well. There is no excuse for the standards of notekeeping and the disarray of results so commonly seen in patients' casenotes. It is also as well to remember the principles of parsimony, because time spent in collecting useless data is time wasted. This applies to all aspects of medicine including questions asked on taking the history from a patient, the examination, and requests for investigations. Some understanding of the principles of the hypothetico-deductive method, and some knowledge of the limitations inherent in the evaluation of tests, are of particular importance in this regard.

Clinical information obtained through conversation with the patient and even from physical examination is often regarded as too 'soft' for scientific respectability, and yet what the patient feels about her predicament is of prime importance. The principles of preservability, objectivity and dimensionality, all of which are regarded as essential features of hard data, do not readily apply to clinical information, although, in truth, they do not apply invariably to data believed to be cast iron. This is also true of histological data which, in the clinical field, is usually regarded as the gold standard. Nevertheless, clinicians should seek to improve objectivity, and composite indices such as the Apgar scale, for assessing the condition of infants, and the Glasgow coma scale add an element of dimensionality and consistency. Quality of life scales, such as the Karnofsky scale for malignancy, could be of increasing importance, particularly in evaluating the real value of treatment. There are many potential pitfalls to be avoided when designing such scales, but this should not deter the steady evolution of this approach which Feinstein calls clinimetrics.

In this book we have looked at potentially important fields such as Bayesian statistics, decision analysis and computer aided diagnosis, in the hope that these sophisticated techniques could be of value in the routine management of patients. Undoubtedly, they have the potential for reducing uncertainty and, in my opinion, the principles on which they are based should be understood by all doctors. However, the widespread implementation of such concepts presents enormous problems, not least of which is the limited time available for decisions to be made. I have not intended to give the impression that they are the answer to all our problems, but there are areas where they could be usefully introduced, particularly when accurate facts are available and decision options are clear cut. Unfortunately, one of the greatest problems in medicine is that accurate information, an essential prerequisite for a correct diagnosis and rational management, is often not available. Perhaps the most useful aspect of these techniques lies in the demands they make for such information, and these demands should help to indicate the type of information which is of prime importance. It is precisely this type of information, required for formal analysis, which can relatively easily be obtained by medical audit, so the current movement in that direction is to be welcomed.

The numerical, statistical, approach does not appeal to many doctors who prefer to understand the root cause of medical problems, managing illness on the basis of pathophysiological reasoning. Whilst this is a desirable aim, there may be so many variables, many of them ill understood or not measureable, that the outcome of management may be predictable only on a statistical basis. In these circumstances the statistical approach is more valid; the use of implausible explanations and false logic can give worse results than acceptance of the random element. As Einhorn[103] pointed out, 'The acceptance of error can lead to less error.' The consistent application of a simple statistical rule may well give better results than the hopeless search for specious connections. Doctors should be prepared to accept and live with this unpalatable truth. They should be clear in their own minds as to where skill is applicable and where chance rules the outcome.

Confusion in this area can lead to inappropriate management with the attendant costs and dangers.

Whilst there is every hope and expectation that the optimum management of medical conditions will become more certain in the future as our knowledge increases, the element of uncertainty will never be eliminated. It seems natural to think in terms of cause and effect, but doctors need to accommodate uncertainty more positively than is currently the case. It has been suggested that we should change from a mechanistic paradigm to one based on probability, but I believe that the two can coexist—much depends upon the type of problem considered and how much is known about it. However, there can be no doubt that medical practice must encompass the problem of uncertainty in a sound comprehensive approach if it is to evolve satisfactorily in the future.

The usual approach to deciding policy when considerable doubt exists is to follow the consensus opinion. In effect, the majority of doctors practise in this way by following the direction laid down by their teachers who, for the most part, convey the current view. The problem is that these views can, and often do, change both rapidly and radically, making continuing education of considerable importance. It may well be true that the shifts of opinions are often based on flimsy evidence, but no doctor should feel comfortable practising without an adequate grasp of current thinking. Achieving this whilst running a busy medical practice is no easy feat; the means by which continuing education is to be attained need to be carefully considered, particularly for family practitioners who cover a wide field of interest. Specialists too have difficulty keeping up in their own field, there being a tendency, as the years go by, to concentrate on the title and summary of a paper rather than on the more important methods section. Incentives for postgraduate education are essential; with sophisticated information technology, increasing use should be made of computer systems which can store up-to-date information in a way that can be accessed easily. The current trend of computer aided diagnostic systems in this direction could prove important.

There is also a place for a consensus view succinctly summarized by a group of experts, and this is becoming more common. The need for a consensus opinion implies differences of views even amongst experts, and there is the potential risk in this approach of what Skrabanek and McCormick[87] call 'the fallacy of the golden mean'. If one view is that $2+2=4$ and another that $2+2=6$, it does not follow that $2+2=5$; the consensus view may not be either sensible or safe. There is also a danger of experts promoting their own interests. Nevertheless, the consensus view is likely to be safer than an individualistic approach as long as it is not regarded as the last word on the topic, otherwise there is a risk of research being stifled. It can be a useful means of pinpointing areas of particular contention.

The acceptance and management of uncertainty can create tension both for the physician and patient. On the part of the physician there can be a feeling of inadequacy leading to a perceived need to do something positive, and on the part of the patient an understandable desire for positive action. This leads to a high rate of unnecessary surgery and the misuse of drugs such as antibiotics and tranquillizers. Both doctors and patients should learn the value of living with uncertainty rather than resolving it in favour of some action which could have detrimental effects on the patient, and economic costs to the community. The desirability of joint participation in medical decisions is unquestionable, particularly as medical decisions become more complex with potential for harm as well as good increasing. The form of this participation depends on the circumstances. Some patients are only too willing to leave the decision to the doctors, but they should at least have the opportunity of discussing the options. Physicians who assume complete autonomy for medical decisions, without giving the patient this opportunity, put themselves in a very difficult ethical position. It may be felt inappropriate to discuss the trade-off between life and disability too explicitly for fear of arousing undue stress, but physicians may not be wise to accept this responsibility.

A point that needs to be considered is whether disclosure of uncertainty is detrimental to the patient. There can be no doubt that not all patients welcome a frank discussion of the possible outcomes of their illness, along with the risks of investigation, and the limitation of treatment. There is a risk of this driving the patient into the arms of quacks who promise certainty and cure however unlikely that may be. But this should not lead to physicians condoning such dishonesty by, similarly, promising the impossible. If, after admitting our limitations, the patient decides to turn to alternative medicine then so be it. Perhaps patients who need a miracle are better off seeking it in some place other than a doctor's surgery. As Katz[104] pointed out, 'In promising more than medicine can deliver, physicians adopt the practice of quacks and are themselves transformed into quacks.'

But does the disclosure of uncertainty diminish the effectiveness of physicians as healers? The placebo effect of a confident physician or an impressive prescription is unquestionable. Whilst most physicians accept and use this, the intellectual discomfort generated may result in the false rationalization of our action. It is as if we are embarrassed by the fact that the effectiveness of many of our practices resides in symbolic power akin to magic. Medicine was born in magic and religion, and the doctor–priest–magician concept seems to reside in the collective unconscious of mankind. Can hope and reassurance be given to patients without resorting to this deception? This may be arguable, but when patients fail to improve with an inappropriately confident approach there is a danger of them feeling disappointed and deceived. Ultimately, a better relationship can be forged by openly discussing uncertainty and participating in a joint venture to find the best approach to their illness.

Little mention has been made in these pages about the organization of health care and ways of optimizing the use of available resources, although some mention of the latter was made in the chapter on decision analysis. With limited resources, and inevitably resources will not be sufficient to take care of all health needs, hard decisions about priorities have to be taken. This poses difficult ethical questions and leads to another aspect of uncertainty. Although I do not believe that these questions should be evaded, this potentially large topic is outside the scope of this book. It is for society to decide where its priorities lie, but the medical profession has an important role to play in clarifying the options. The techniques mentioned in this book are a starting point for rational analysis of options.

One further difficulty faced by the inexperienced doctor is in knowing whether his uncertainty arises because of his own lack of knowledge, or because the relevant knowledge is simply not available. There is no simple answer to this dilemma, but, in the best tradition of medicine, I can assure the young doctor that the problem eases with time as experience and confidence increase. It is, nevertheless, as well to bear in mind that all of us are undergraduates in the school of experience; there is a danger of becoming a public menace to think otherwise. It is true that an apparently knowledgeable and authoritative physician can not only get away with the most flagrant imprecision, vagueness and inconsistency, but he can also be praised for it. This is not, however, a course I find attractive or would recommend. Respect for authority should be tempered with a little circumspection. Even the written word is not above suspicion. Many errors are promulgated from one textbook to another. The belief that spinach is a rich source of iron is one such error which arose from a decimal point being put in the wrong place by the original investigator.

The legal responsibility for unfortunate outcomes is a further source of worry for all doctors. When dealing with uncertain outcomes, it is inevitable that sometimes the correct decision can lead to a bad outcome. Whilst patients may have difficulty accepting this, doctors must learn to live with it and, by and large, the legal position in these circumstances would be in favour of the doctor. Whilst the likelihood of an unfortunate outcome may be reduced by further investigation or expensive management, there comes a point where decreasing the uncertainty can put the patient at greater risk. This may be true when more invasive investigations are required and with defensive surgical procedures such as 'routine' caesarean sections. The legal profession and society must appreciate that defensive medicine is not only expensive but it can also be unsafe. When a doctor is likely to be sued for doing too little rather than too much, there will be an inevitable trend towards expensive health care which will not necessarily benefit the health of the individual or the community. With private health care, defensive medicine is also profitable medicine so doctors may not resist this trend. Politicians should appreciate this dilemma if they are concerned with optimizing the use of available resources.

Respect for authority tends to be the basis of most medical education, but the student would be wise to question even long established practices. This must not stop him acquiring a working knowledge of current beliefs, but he should not accept them as incontestable facts. It is only by having doubts that the practice of medicine will progress. Uncertainty and doubt may seem weak foundations on which to base medical practice, but the alternative, unthinking didacticism, is unacceptable. As Harold Macmillan put it, 'To be uncertain is uncomfortable, but to be certain is ridiculous.' It is only by accepting uncertainty and yet seeking ways to reduce it that medicine can move forward.

References

1. Medawar, P. B. Induction and intuition in scientific thought. *Memoirs of the American Philosophical Society* 1969; **75**: 5577.1.
2. Hawking, S. *A Brief History of Time*. London: Bantam Press. 1988.
3. Campbell, E. J. M., Scadding, J. G. and Roberts, R. S. The concept of disease. *British Medical Journal* 1979; **ii**: 757–762.
4. Reznek, L. *The Nature of Disease*. London: Routledge and Kegan Paul. 1987.
5. Scadding, J. G. Diagnosis: The clinician and the computer. *Lancet* 1961; Oct. 21: 877–882.
6. Jennings, D. Perforated peptic ulcer. Changes in age incidence and sex distribution in the last 150 years. *Lancet* 1940; **i**: 395–398 and 444–447.
7. With, C. *The Clinical Picture, Diagnosis and Treatment of Gastric Ulcer* (in Danish). Copenhagen: Gyldendal. 1881.
8. Bronowski, J. *The Common Sense of Science*. Penguin Books. 1960. p. 38.
9. Russell, B. *The Problems of Philosophy*. Oxford: Oxford University Press. 1912.
10. Whewell, W. *The Philosophy of the Inductive Sciences*, Vol. 2. London: Parker. 1840.
11. Popper, K. R. *The Logic of Scientific Discovery*. London: Hutchinson. 1959.
12. Kuhn, T. S. *The Structure of Scientific Revolutions*. The University of Chicago Press. 1962.
13. Black, D. *An Anthology of False Antitheses*. London: Nuffield Provincial Hospital Trust. 1984.
14. Thomas, K. B. General practice consultations: Is there any point in being positive? *British Medical Journal* 1987; **294**: 1200–1202.
15. Skrabanek, P. and McCormick, J. *Follies and Fallacies in Medicine*. Glasgow: The Tarragon Press. 1989. p. 70.

16. Haynes, R. B., Sackett, D. L., Wayne Taylor, D., Gibson, E. S. and Johnson, A. L. Increased absenteeism from work after detection and labelling of hypertensive patients. *New England Journal of Medicine* 1978; **299**: 741–744.
17. Feinstein, A. R. The chagrin factor and qualitative decision analysis. *Archives of Internal Medicine* 1985; **145**: 1257–1259.
18. Kassirer, J. P. Sounding board—our stubborn quest for diagnostic certainty—a case of excessive testing. *New England Journal of Medicine* 1989; **320**: 1489–1491.
19. Inhelder, B. and Piaget, J. *The Growth of Logical Thinking from Childhood to Adolescence*. London: Routledge and Kegan Paul. 1958.
20. Barrows, H. S., Norman, G. R., Neufield, V. R. and Feightner, J. W. The clinical reasoning of randomly selected physicians in general medical practice. *Clinical and Investigative Medicine* 1982; **5**: 49–55.
21. Elstein, A. S., Shulman, L. S. and Sprafka, S. A. *Medical Problem Solving: An Analysis of Clinical Reasoning*. Cambridge, Mass: Harvard University Press. 1978.
22. Kassirer, J. P. and Gorry, A. Clinical problem solving: A behavioural analysis. *Annals of Internal Medicine* 1978; **89**: 245–255.
23. Leaper, D. J., Gill, P. W., Staniland, J. R., Horrocks, J. C. and De Dombal, F. T. Clinical diagnostic process: an analysis. *British Medical Journal* 1973; **iii**: 569–574.
24. Balla, J. I. The use of critical cues and prior probability in decision making. *Methods of Information in Medicine* 1982; **21**: 9–14.
25. Eddy, D. M. and Clanton, C. H. The art of diagnosis: solving the clinical pathological exercise. *New England Journal of Medicine* 1982; **306**: 1263–1268.
26. Kozielecki, J. A model for diagnostic problem solving. *Acta Psychologica* 1972; **36**: 370–380.
27. Gorry, G. A., Pauker, S. G. and Schwartz, W. B. The diagnostic importance of the normal finding. *New England Journal of Medicine* 1978; **298**: 486–489.
28. Gale, J. and Marsden, P. *Medical Diagnosis; From Student to Clinician*. Oxford: Oxford Medical Publications. 1983.
29. Norman, G. R., Barrows, H. S., Neufeld, V. R. and Feigntner, J. W. A data base for analysis of the process of clinical problem solving. *Proceedings, Medinfo*. Amsterdam: North Holland. Shires and Wolf. 1977.
30. Balla, J. I., Rothert, M., Greenbaum, D. and Black, N. A. Diagnostic cues in gastroenterology. *Australian and New Zealand Journal of Medicine* 1983; **13**: 469–77.
31. Balla, J. I., Elstein, A. S. and Gates, P. Effect of prevalence and

test diagnosticity upon clinical judgement of probability. *Methods of Information in Medicine* 1983; **22**: 25–28.

32. Hampton, J. R., Harrison, M. J. G., Mitchell, J. R. A., Prichard, J. S. and Seymour, C. Relative contributions of history taking, physical examination and laboratory investigations to diagnosis and management of medical outpatients. *British Medical Journal* 1975; **ii**: 486–489.
33. Hoffbrand, B. I. Away with the system review: A plea for parsimony. *British Medical Journal* 1989; **298**: 817–819.
34. Gross, F. The emperor's clothes syndrome. *New England Journal of Medicine* 1971; **285**: 863.
35. Fletcher, C. M. Clinical diagnosis of pulmonary emphysema; experimental study. *Proceedings of the Royal Society of Medicine* 1952; **45**: 577–584.
36. Garland, L. H. Studies of the accuracy of diagnostic procedures. *American Journal of Roentgenology* 1959; **82**: 25–38.
37. Koran, L. M. The reliability of clinical methods, data and judgement. *New England Journal of Medicine* 1975; **293**: 642–646.
38. Koran, L. M. The reliability of clinical methods, data and judgement. *New England Journal of Medicine* 1975; **293**: 695–702.
39. Cochrane, A. L. and Garland, L. H. Observer error in interpretation of chest films; international investigations. *Lancet* 1952; **ii**: 505–509.
40. Feinstein, A. R. A bibliography of publications on observer variability. *Journal of Chronic Diseases* 1985; **38**: 619–632.
41. Sandler, D. A., Duncan, J. S., Ward, P. et al. Diagnosis of deep vein thrombosis; comparison of clinical evaluation, ultrasound, plethysmography and venoscan with X-ray venogram. *Lancet* 1984; **ii**: 716–718.
42. Hamm, R. M. Clinical intuition and clinical analysis; expertise and the cognitive continuum. *Professional Judgement* (Ed. Dowie, J. and Elstein, A.), Chapter 3. Cambridge University Press. 1988.
43. Hammond, K. R., McClelland, G. H. and Mumpower, J. *Human Judgement and Decision Making*. New York: Hemisphere. 1980.
44. Dreyfus, H. L., and Dreyfus, S. E. *Mind Over Machine: The Power of Human Intuition and Expertise in the Era of the Computer*. Oxford: Blackwell. 1986.
45. Ledley, R. S. and Lusted, L. B. Reasoning foundations of medical diagnosis. *Science* 1959; **130**: 9–21.
46. Gibson, R. S. and Beller, G. A. Should exercise electrocardiographic testing be replaced by radioisotope methods? *Cardiovascular Clinics* 1983; **13**: 1–31.
47. Yerushalmy, J. Statistical problems in assessing methods of medical diagnosis, with special reference to X-ray techniques. *Public Health Report* 1947; **62**: 1432–1449.

48. Wulff, H. R. *Rational Diagnosis and Treatment: An Introduction to Clinical Decision Making*. Oxford: Blackwell Scientific Publications. 1976.
49. McNeil, B. J., Keller, E. and Adelstein, J. Primer on certain elements of medical decision making. *New England Journal of Medicine* 1975; **293**: 211–215.
50. Noe, D. E. *The Logic of Laboratory Medicine*. Baltimore: Urban and Schwarzenberg. 1985.
51. Fryback, D. G. Bayes' Theorem and conditional non independence of Data in medical diagnosis. *Computers and Biomedical Research* 1978; **11**: 423–434.
52. Spiegelhalter, D. J. Statistical aids in clinical decision making. *Statistician* 1982; **31**: 19–36.
53. Spiegelhalter, D. J. and Knill-Jones, R. P. Statistical and knowledge based approaches to clinical decisions. *Journal of the Royal Statistical Society (Series A)* 1984; **147**: 35–77.
54. Seymour, D. G., Green, M. and Vaz, F. G. Making better decisions: construction of clinical scoring systems by the Spiegelhalter-Knill Jones approach. *British Medical Journal* 1990; **300**: 223–226.
55. Dolan, J. G., Bordley, D. R. and Mushlin, A. I. An evaluation of clinicians subjective prior probability estimates. *Medical Decision Making* 1986; **6**: 216–223.
56. Turing, A. M. Computing machinery and intelligence. *Mind* **59** no. 236.
57. Penrose, R. *The Emperor's New Mind*. Oxford: Oxford University Press. 1989.
58. Reggia, J. A. and Tuhrim, S. (eds.) *Computers and Medicine: Computer Assisted Medical Decision Making*, Vol. 1 and 2. New York: Springer-Verlag. 1985.
59. Bleich, H. Computer-based consultation. *American Journal of Medicine* 1972; **53**: 285–291.
60. Jelliffe, R., Buell, J. and Kalaba, R. Reduction of digitalis toxicity by computer assisted glycoside dosage regimens. *Annals of Internal Medicine* 1972; **77**: 891–906.
61. De Dombal, F. T., Leaper, D. J., Staniland, J. R., McCann, A. P. and Horrocks, J. C. Computer aided diagnosis of acute abdominal pain. *British Medical Journal* 1972; **ii**: 9–13.
62. Adams, I. D. et al. Computer aided diagnosis of abdominal pain: a multicentre study. *British Medical Journal* 1986; **293**: 800–804.
63. Davis, R., Buchanan, B. and Shortliffe, E. Production rules as a representation for a knowledge-based consultation programme. *Artificial Intelligence* 1977; **8**: 15–45.
64. Weiss, S., Kulikowski, C. and Safir, A. Glaucoma consultation by computer. *Computers in Biological Medicine* 1978; **8**: 25–40.

65. Kunz, J. et al. A Physiological Rule-Based System for Interpreting Pulmonary Function Test Results, HPP-78-19. Department of Computer Science Stanford University. 1978.
66. Weed, L. L. and Hertzberg, R. Problem solving: What's the best combination of man and machine. *Computer Medical Update* 1984; 2: 4–16.
67. Miller, R. A., Pople, H. E. and Myers, J. D. INTERNIST I. An experimental computer based diagnostic consultant for general internal medicine. *New England Journal of Medicine* 1982; **307**: 468–476.
68. Mittal, S., Chandrasekaren, B. and Smith, J. Overview of MDX—a System for Medical Diagnoses. *Proceedings of the Third Symposium of Computer Application in Medical Care.* IEEE. 1979. pp. 34–46.
69. Catanzarite, V. and Greenburg, A. Neurologist. A Computer Programme for Diagnoses in Neurology. *Proceedings of the Third Symposium of Computer Applications in Medical Care.* IEEE. 1979. pp. 64–72.
70. Bakwin, H. Pseudodoxia pediatrica. *New England Journal of Medicine* 1945; **232**: 691–697.
71. Sox, H. C. Jr, Blatt, M. R., Higgins, M. C. and Marton, K. I. *Medical Decision Making.* Boston: Butterworth. 1988.
72. Kassirer, J. P., Moskowitz, A. J., Lau, J. and Pauker, S. G. Decision analysis: a progress report. *Annals of Internal Medicine* 1987; **106**: 275–291.
73. Beck, J. R., Kassirer, J. P. and Pauker, S. G. A convenient approximation of life expectancy. *American Journal of Medicine* 1982; **73**: 883–888.
74. Mooney, G. and Olsen, J. A. *Providing Health Care* (Ed. McQuire, A., Fenn, P. and Mayhew, K.), Chapter 5. Oxford: Oxford University Press. 1991. pp. 120–140.
75. Doubilet, I., Weinstein, M. C. and McNeil, B. J. Use and misuse of the term 'cost effective' in medicine. *New England Journal of Medicine* 1986; **314**: 253–255.
76. Weinstein, M. C. and Stason, W. B. Foundations of cost effectiveness analysis for health and medical practices. *New England Journal of Medicine* 1977; **296**: 716–721.
77. Eraker, S. A. and Politser, P. How decisions are reached: physicians and patients. *Annals of Internal Medicine* 1982; **97**: 262–268.
78. McNeil, B. J., Pauker, S. G., Sox, H. C. and Tversky, A. On the elicitation of preferences for alternative therapies. *New England Journal of Medicine* 1982; **306**: 1259–1262.
79. Moskowitz, A. J., Kuipers, B. J. and Kassirer, J. P. Dealing with uncertainty, risks and tradeoffs in clinical decisions. *Annals of Internal Medicine* 1988; **108**: 435–449.

80. Hershey, J. C. and Baron J. Clinical reasoning and cognitive processes. *Medical Decision Making* 1987; **7**: 203–211.

81. Schwartz, W. B. Sounding board—decision analysis. *New England Journal of Medicine* 1979; **300**: 556–559.

82. Kassirer, J. P. and Pauker, S. G. The toss up. *New England Journal of Medicine* 1981; **305**: 1467–1469.

83. Clarke, J. R. Decision making in surgical practice. *World Journal of Surgery* 1989; **13**: 245–251.

84. Howson, C. and Urbach, P. *Scientific Reasoning: The Bayesian Approach*. Illinois: Open Court Publishing Company. 1989.

85. Blackwell, B., Bloomsfield, S. S. and Buncher, C. R. Demonstration to medical students of placebo response and non-drug factors. *Lancet* 1972; **i**: 1279–1282.

86. Cobb, L. A., Thomas, G. J., Dillard, D. H., Merindino, K. A. and Bruce, R. A. An evaluation of internal mammary artery ligation by a double-blind technic. *New England Jornal of Medicine* 1959; **260**: 1115–1118.

87. Skrabanek, P. and McCormick, J. *Follies and Fantasies in Medicine*. Glasgow: The Tarragon Press. 1989. p. 12.

88. Sackett, D. L. Bias in analytic research. *Journal of Chronic Diseases* 1979; **32**: 51–63.

89. Feinstein, A. R. An additional basic science for clinical medicine. II. The limitations of randomized trials. *Annals of Internal Medicine* 1983; **99**: 544–550.

90. Sterling, T. D. Publication decisions and their possible effects on inferences drawn from tests of significance or vice versa. *Journal of American Statistical Association* 1959; **54**: 30–34.

91. Begg, C. B. and Berlin, J. A. Publication bias: a problem in interpreting medical data. *Journal of the Royal Statistical Society A* 1988; **151**: 419–463.

92. Coursol, A. and Wagner, E. E. Effect of positive findings on submission and acceptance rates—a note on meta analysis bias. *Professional Psychology* 1986; **17**: 136–137.

93. Sacks, H. S., Chalmers, T. C. and Smith, H. Sensitivity and specificity of clinical trials: randomized versus historical controls. *Archives of Internal Medicine* 1983; **143**: 753–755.

94. Davidson, R. A. Source of funding and outcome of clinical trials. *Journal of General Internal Medicine* 1986; **1**: 155–158.

95. Ward, M. J. Clinical trials in acute severe asthma: are Type II errors important? *Thorax* 1986; **41**: 824–829.

96. Fortney, J. A., Potts, M. and Bonhomme, M. Invasive cancer and combined oral contraceptives. *British Medical Journal* 1985; **290**: 1587.

97. Glass, G. V. Primary, secondary and meta analysis of research. *Educational Research* 1976; **5**: 3–8.

98. Sack, H. S., Berrier, J., Reitman, D., Ancona-Berk, V. A. and Chalmers, T. C. Meta analysis of randomized controlled trials. *New England Journal of Medicine* 1987; **316**: 450–455.

99. Thacker, S. B. Meta analysis—a qualitative approach to research integration. *Journal of the American Medical Association* 1988; **259**(11): 1685–1689.

100. Collins, R., Yusuf, S. and Peto, R. Overview of randomized trials of diuretics in pregnancy. *British Medical Journal* 1985; **290**: 17–23.

101. Mantel, N. and Haenszel, W. Statistical aspects of the analysis of data from retrospective studies of disease. *Journal of the National Cancer Institute* 1959; **22**: 719–748.

102. Thompson, S. G. and Pocock, S. J. Can meta analyses be trusted? *Lancet* 1991; **338**: 1127–1130.

103. Einhorn, H. J. Accepting error to make less error. *Journal of Personality Assessment* 1986; **50**: 387–95.

104. Katz, J. Why doctors don't disclose uncertainty. *Hastings Centre Report* 1984; **14**: 35–44.

Index

Index compiled by Liza Weinkove